BASICS OF CANCER CHEMOTHERAPY

3rd Edition

By
Ellen Carr, RN, MSN and
Judith A. Killman, BSN, MA, MS

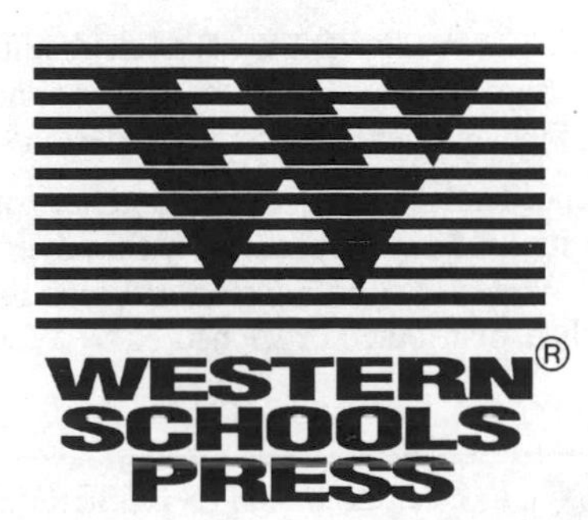

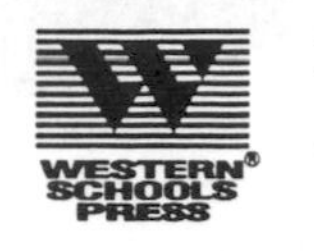

21 Bristol Drive
South Easton, MA 02375
1-800-618-1670

ABOUT THE AUTHORS

Ellen Carr, RN, MSN, is a clinical nurse specialist for Pancretec, a subsidiary of Abbott Laboratories in San Diego, California. Earlier, she was the oncology clinical nurse specialist at Green Hospital of Scripps Clinic and Research Foundation in La Jolla, California. She holds a master of science degree in oncology nursing from the MGH Institute of Health Professions in Boston and a bachelor of science degree in journalism from the University of Colorado.

Judith A. Killman, BSN, MA, MS, is a Navy Nurse Corps officer stationed at the Naval Hospital San Diego. She is the head of the Ambulatory Maternal Child Nursing Department. LCDR Killman has extensive experience in clinical oncology nursing and was instrumental in developing a chemotherapeutic agent certification course for nurses caring for oncology patients.

ABOUT THE SUBJECT MATTER EXPERT

Cindy Jones, RN, MS, OCN, has more than 11 years experience in adult medical oncology. She has developed numerous staff and patient educational programs. She has facilitated support groups for cancer patients and their families and has been an instructor on oncologic topics on the local, state, and national level. She is currently an oncology clinical nurse specialist for the Veterans Affairs Medical Center in San Diego, California, where she initiated the Cancer Symptom Management Clinic.

ABOUT THE REVIEWER

Rebecca S. Finley, PharmD, MS is currently Head, Section of Pharmacy Services at the University of Maryland Cancer Center. She also holds the appointments of Pharmacy School Associate Professor in the Department of Pharmacy Practice and Science at the University of Maryland and Associate Professor of Oncology at the University of Maryland Cancer Center and School of Medicine. She received her BS and PharmD degrees from the University of Cincinnati and her MS in Institutional Pharmacy from the University of Maryland. She is currently President-elect of the American Society of Hospital Pharmacists and has served as Chairperson of the ASHP Special Interest Group in Oncology, and is a Past President of Maryland Society of Hospital Pharmacists and has served on its Board of Directors. Dr. Finley served on the Agency for Health Care Policy and Research Cancer Pain Guideline expert panel, and also serves on the steering committee of *Cancer Pain Strategies for Maryland-The Maryland Cancer Pain Initiative.*

Copy Editor: Barbara L. Halliburton, PhD

Graphics Coordinator: Kathy Johnson

ISBN: 1-878025-71-6

IMPORTANT: Read these instructions *BEFORE* proceeding!

Enclosed with your course book you will find the FasTrax® answer sheet. Use this form to answer all the final exam questions that appear in this course book. If you are completing more than one course, be sure to write your answers on the appropriate answer sheet. Full instructions and complete grading details are printed on the FasTrax instruction sheet, also enclosed with your order. Please review them before starting. *If you are mailing your answer sheet(s) to Western Schools, we recommend you make a copy as a backup.*

ABOUT THIS COURSE

A "Pretest" is provided with each course to test your current knowledge base regarding the subject matter contained within this course. Your "Final Exam" is a multiple choice examination. **You will find the exam questions at the end of each chapter.** Some smaller hour courses include the exam at the end of the book.

In the event the course has less than 100 questions, mark your answers to the questions in the course book and leave the remaining answer boxes on the FasTrax answer sheet blank. **Use a black pen to fill in your answer sheet.**

A PASSING SCORE

You must score 70% or better in order to pass this course and receive your Certificate of Completion. Should you fail to achieve the required score, we will send you an additional FasTrax answer sheet so that you may make a second attempt to pass the course. Western Schools will allow you three chances to pass the same course...*at no extra charge!* After three failed attempts to pass the same course, your file will be closed.

RECORDING YOUR HOURS

Please monitor the time it takes to complete this course using the handy log sheet on the other side of this page. See below for transferring study hours to the course evaluation.

COURSE EVALUATIONS

In this course book you will find a short evaluation about the course you are soon to complete. This information is vital to providing the school with feedback on this course. The course evaluation answer section is in the lower right hand corner of the FasTrax answer sheet marked "Evaluation" with answers marked 1–25. Your answers are important to us, please take five minutes to complete the evaluation.

On the back of the FasTrax instruction sheet there is additional space to make any comments about the course, the school, and suggested new curriculum. Please mail the FasTrax instruction sheet, with your comments, back to Western Schools in the envelope provided with your course order.

TRANSFERRING STUDY TIME

Upon completion of the course, transfer the total study time from your log sheet to question #25 in the Course Evaluation. The answers will be in ranges, please choose the proper hour range that best represents your study time. You MUST log your study time under question #25 on the course evaluation.

EXTENSIONS

You have 2 years from the date of enrollment to complete this course. A six (6) month extension may be purchased. If after 30 months from the original enrollment date you do not complete the course, *your file will be closed and no certificate can be issued.*

CHANGE OF ADDRESS?

In the event you have moved during the completion of this course please call our student services department at 1-800-618-1670 and we will update your file.

A GUARANTEE YOU'LL GIVE HIGH HONORS TO

If any continuing education course fails to meet your expectations or if you are not satisfied in any manner, for any reason, you may return it for an exchange or a refund (less shipping and handling) within 30 days. Software, video and audio courses must be returned unopened.

Thank you for enrolling at Western Schools!

WESTERN SCHOOLS
P.O. Box 1930
Brockton, MA 02303
(800) 618-1670

Basics of Cancer Chemotherapy

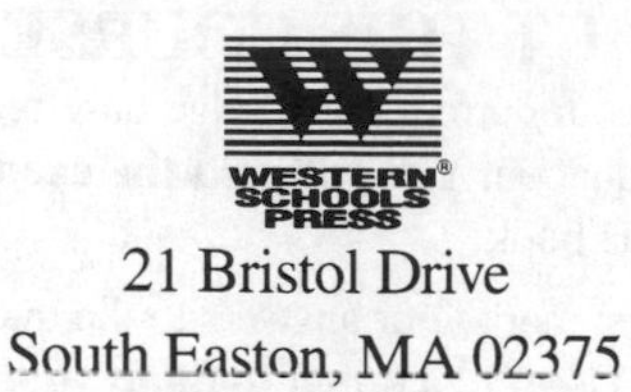

21 Bristol Drive
South Easton, MA 02375

Please use this log to total the number of hours you spend reading the text and taking the final examination (use 50-min hours).

Date	Hours Spent
____________	____________
____________	____________
____________	____________
____________	____________
____________	____________
____________	____________
____________	____________
____________	____________
____________	____________
____________	____________
____________	____________
____________	____________
____________	____________
____________	____________
TOTAL	

Please log your study hours with submission of your final exam. To log your study time, fill in the appropriate circle under question 25 of the FasTrax® answer sheet under the "Evaluation" section.

Please choose the answer that represents the total study hours it took you to complete this 15 hour course.

A. less than 10 hours
B. 10–13 hours
C. 14–17 hours
D. greater than 17 hours

BASICS OF CANCER CHEMOTHERAPY

WESTERN SCHOOLS' NURSING
CONTINUING EDUCATION EVALUATION

Instructions: Mark your answers to the following questions with a black pen on the "Evaluation" section of your FasTrax® answer sheet provided with this course. You should not return this sheet. Please use the scale below to rate the following statements:

A Agree Strongly
B Agree Somewhat
C Disagree Somewhat
D Disagree Strongly

The course content met the following education objectives:

1. Described why chemotherapy is the treatment of choice for some malignancies and stated the criteria used to measure the effectiveness of the treatment.
2. Discussed the phases of the cell cycle and why chemotherapy can affect or destroy cancer cells.
3. Discussed classifications of chemotherapeutic agents and how these agents act on malignant and normal cells.
4. Described principles of safe administration of chemotherapeutic agents.
5. Named specific chemotherapeutic agents, how they are given, and their side effects.
6. Described side effects of chemotherapy and how they might be managed.
7. Described additional approaches to chemotherapy.
8. The content of this course was relevant to the objectives.
9. This offering met my professional education needs.
10. The information in this offering is relevant to my professional work setting.
11. The course was generally well written and the subject matter explained thoroughly? (If no please explain on the back of the FasTrax instruction sheet.)
12. The content of this course was appropriate for home study.
13. The final examination was well written and at an appropriate level for the content of the course.

Please complete the following research questions in order to help us better meet your educational needs. Pick the ONE answer which is most appropriate.

14. How did you fulfill the majority of your CE requirement the time just before this Western Schools order?
    - A. Western Schools
    - B. Another home study provider
    - C. Seminars or in-house lectures
    - D. No previous occasion
15. Which answer best describes the portion of your total Continuing Education hours that were completed by home study during your last renewal?
    - A. All
    - B. Half to more than half
    - C. Less than half
    - D. None

16. Are you reimbursed for your Continuing Education hours, and if so, by what dollar percentage?
    A. All
    B. Half to more than half
    C. Less than half
    D. None
17. What is your work status?
    A. Full-time employment
    B. Part-time employment
    C. Per diem/Temporary employment
    D. Inactive/Retired
18. For your LAST renewal did you take more Continuing Education contact hours than required by your state, if so, how many?
    A. 1–15 hours
    B. 16–30 hours
    C. 31 or more hours
    D. No, I only take the state required minimum
19. Do you usually exceed the contact hours required for your state license renewal, if so, why?
    A. Yes, I have more than one state license
    B. Yes, to meet additional special association Continuing Education requirements
    C. Yes, for professional self-interest/cross-training
    D. No, I only take the state required minimum
20. What nursing shift do you most commonly work?
    A. Morning Shift (Any shift starting after 3:00am or before 11:00am)
    B. Day/Afternoon Shift (Any shift starting after 11:00am or before 7:00pm)
    C. Night Shift (Any shift starting after 7:00pm or before 3:00am)
    D. I work rotating shifts
21. What was the SINGLE most important reason you chose this course?
    A. Low Price
    B. New or Newly revised course
    C. High interest/Required course topic
    D. Number of Contact Hours Needed
22. Where do you work? (If your place of employment is not listed below, please leave this question blank.)
    A. Hospital
    B. Medical Clinic/Group Practice/ HMO/Office setting
    C. Long Term Care/Rehabilitation Facility/Nursing Home
    D. Home Health Care Agency
23. Which field do you specialize in?
    A. Medical/Surgical
    B. Geriatrics
    C. Pediatrics/Neonatal
    D. Other
24. For your last renewal, how many months BEFORE your license expiration date did your order your course materials?
    A. 1–3 months
    B. 4–6 months
    C. 7–12 months
    D. Greater than 12 months
25. **PLEASE LOG YOUR STUDY HOURS WITH SUBMISSION OF YOUR FINAL EXAM.** Please choose which best represents the total study hours it took to complete this 15 hour course.
    A. less than 10 hours
    B. 10–13 hours
    C. 14–17 hours
    D. greater than 17 hours

TABLE OF CONTENTS

Evaluation
Course Objectives
Pre-test
Introduction
***Chapter 1* Overview** **1**
History 1
Vocabulary 2
Effectiveness of Chemotherapy 2
Goals of Chemotherapy 3
Tumor Response Criteria 4
Exam Questions 5
***Chapter 2* Biology of Chemotherapy** **7**
Cell Cycle 7
Birthrate of Cells 8
Cell Kill Hypothesis 11
Exam Questions 13
***Chapter 3* Drug Classifications** **15**
Alkylating Agents 15
Antimetabolites 17
Antitumor Antibiotics 17
Plant Alkaloids 17
Nitrosoureas 18
Hormones 18
Miscellaneous Agents 18
Exam Questions 19
***Chapter 4* Administration of Chemotherapeutic Agents** **21**
Knowledge About the Patient 21
Knowledge and Skills Needed to Administer the Agents 22
Education of the Patient 37
Exam Questions 39
***Chapter 5* Selected Chemotherapeutic Agents** **41**
Bleomycin (Blenoxane) 41
Busulfan (Myleran) 42
Carmustine (BCNU) 42
Cisplatin (Platinum, Platinol) 43
Cyclophosphamide (Cytoxan, CTX) 44

Cytarabine (ARA-C, Cytosar-U, Cytosine, Arabinoside) .44
Dacarbazine (DTIC, Imidazole, Carboximide) .45
Dactinomycin (Actinomycin D, Cosmegen) .45
Daunorubicin (Daunomycin, Rubidomycin, Cerubidine) .46
Doxorubicin Hydrochloride (Adriamycin) .46
Etoposide (VP-16, VePesid) .47
Flurouracil (Flourouracil, Adricil, 5FU) .47
Floxuridine (FUDR) .48
Hydroxyurea (Hydrea) .48
Ifosfamide (IFEX, Isophosphamide) .49
L-Asparaginase (Elspar) .49
Lomustine (CCNU, CEENU) .50
Mechlorethamine (Nitrogen Mustard, Mustargen, HN2) .50
Megestrol (Megace, Pallace) .51
Methotrexate (Mexate, MTX) .51
Mitomycin (Mutamycin) .52
Mitoxantrone (Novantrone, DHAD) .52
Plicamycin (Mithramycin, Mithracin) .53
Prednisone (Deltasone, Orasone) .53
Procarbazine (Matulane) .54
6-Mercaptopurine (Purinethol, 6MP) .54
Tamoxifen (Nolvadex) .54
Thiotepa (Triethylene, Thiophosphoramide) .55
Vinblastine (Velban, VLB) .55
Vincristine (Oncovin, VCR) .56
Exam Questions .557
***Chapter 6* Management of Patients .59**
Bone Marrow Suppression .60
Stomatitis .62
Nausea and Vomiting .64
Alopecia .64
Anorexia and Weight Loss .66
Constipation .66
Diarrhea .67
Nephrotoxic Effects .67
Secondary Malignancy .67
Gonadal Dysfunction .67
Extravasation .68
Anaphylaxis .69
Pain .71

Psychosocial Concerns .71
Exam Questions .72
***Chapter 7* Developments in Chemotherapy .75**
Combination Therapy .75
New Drugs .77
Dosages .79
Adjuvant Chemotherapy .79
Colony Stimulating Factors .79
Prevention .80
Clinical Trials .80
Delivery Options: Chemotherapy Administration Away from the Hospital .81
Exam Questions .82
Bibliography .83
Suggested Reading List .85
Glossary .87
***Appendix A* Venous Access Devices .89**
Vascular Access Devices .90
Long-Term Catheters .91
Implanted Ports .92
Implanted Pumps (Medtronic) .93
Implanted Pumps (INFUSAID) .94
PICC Line .95
***Appendix B* Performance Status Scales .97**
Index
Pre-test Key

COURSE OBJECTIVES

At the end of this course, each participant will be able to

1. Describe the goals for using chemotherapy and when this treatment is indicated.
2. Explain the action of two chemotherapeutic agents in relation to the cell cycle.
3. Identify two chemotherapeutic agents according to the classification of such agents.
4. List two chemotherapeutic agents that are considered vesicants and describe three ways to avoid extravasation.
5. Describe the agents used in two combination chemotherapy treatments.
6. Explain the term "nadir" and state how a nadir affects two chemotherapy treatments.
7. Identify three developments in chemotherapy treatments.
8. Identify five aspects of administering chemotherapy safely and correctly.
9. Describe six routes of administration of chemotherapy.
10. Identify and describe three side effects associated with chemotherapy and how they might be managed.

PRE-TEST

Begin by taking the pre-test. Compare your answers on the pre-test to the answer key (located in the back of the book). Circle those test items that you missed. The pre-test answer key indicates the chapters where the content of that question is discussed.

Next, read each chapter. Focus special attention on the chapters where you made incorrect answer choices. Study questions are provided at the end of each chapter so that you can assess your progress and understanding of the material.

1. What are the primary goals of chemotherapy?

   a. Cure and control the growth of tumors to relieve symptoms when a cure is not possible
   b. Control tumor growth and boost immune system
   c. Expose cancer and relieve symptoms
   d. Stimulate tumor growth and boost immune system

2. Which of the following drugs act on all phases of the cell cycle?

   a. Vinblastine, procarbazine, 5FU
   b. Cisplatin, BCNU, doxorubicin
   c. Prednisone, methotrexate, CCNU
   d. Bleomycin, vincristine, busulfan

3. Interventions that prevent or minimize extravasation of chemotherapeutic agents include

   a. Monitoring the patient throughout administration
   b. Infusing the agent rapidly and flushing the vein frequently with normal saline
   c. Ensuring the patency of the vein by assessing for an adequate blood return 30 minutes after administration of the agent
   d. Giving the infusion at 1-hour intervals if discomfort at the infusion site is noted

4. The nurse's role in administering chemotherapeutic agents includes

   a. Administering chemotherapy before checking the laboratory data
   b. Giving the agents in a rushed, hurried environment
   c. Administering chemotherapy before establishing informed consent
   d. Teaching the patient what to expect during and after administration

5. What should the nurse do if a small amount of a nonvesicant agent infiltrates during its administration?

   a. Give epinephrine.
   b. Discontinue the infusion and restart the injection at a different site.
   c. Leave the needle in place and aspirate as much of the residual medication as possible.
   d. Complete the injection.

6. Patients receiving a drug known to decrease the number of platelets should be instructed to report which of the following findings immediately?

   a. Shortness of breath
   b. Increased bruising
   c. Change of hair color
   d. Fever

7. A common combination for chemotherapy is

   a. ZZN
   b. LQR
   c. MRI
   d. CHOP

8. Megace® is classified as

   a. An alkylating agent
   b. An antimetabolite
   c. A hormone
   d. A nitrosurea

9. Constipation is a common complication of patients receiving which of the following chemotherapeutic agents?

   a. 5FU
   b. Vincristine
   c. Methotrexate
   d. ARA-C

10. Treatment of which cancer has been associated with secondary malignancies?

    a. Melanoma
    b. Hodgkin's disease
    c. Glioblastomas
    d. Lung cancer

INTRODUCTION

Chemotherapy is one method or modality to treat patients who have cancer. Although the term chemotherapy is used generically to refer to the use of drugs in cancer treatment, it actually means treatment of any disease with chemical agents. Along with chemotherapy, the other ways to treat cancer patients are radiation therapy, surgery, and immunotherapy. How a tumor is treated depends on what type of tumor it is and where the tumor is located.

The intent of this book is to familiarize you with reasons for using chemotherapy as a sole treatment for cancer or in conjunction with the other standard methods of treatment. In some cases, tumor cells are killed more efficiently when a combination of treatments is used. This book concentrates on the rationale behind using chemotherapy, profiles of commonly used drugs, and trends in chemotherapeutic treatments.

This book is not intended to provide a curriculum to certify you to give chemotherapy. Certification courses require more detail and hands-on instruction, and appropriate courses are available through hospitals and colleges. Many excellent references and study guides exist for those who plan to give chemotherapeutic agents regularly. Nevertheless, this book is a thorough, practical overview of chemotherapy as a treatment for cancer. Cancer is the second most common cause of death in the United States; thus, a working knowledge of its treatment is crucial for any health professional in practice today.

CHAPTER 1

OVERVIEW

CHAPTER OBJECTIVE

After completing this chapter, you will be able to describe why chemotherapy is the treatment of choice for some malignancies and state the criteria used to measure the effectiveness of the treatment.

LEARNING OBJECTIVES

After reading this chapter, the reader will be able to

1. Define three basic terms referring to chemotherapy in cancer.
2. Indicate two treatment goals of chemotherapy.
3. Identify three tumors that have been known to respond to chemotherapy.
4. Indicate three criteria used to analyze the effectiveness of chemotherapy.

In providing a course overview, this chapter gives a brief history of how chemotherapeutic treatments began, an initial review of the vocabulary of cancer, effectiveness of chemotherapy as a cancer treatment, goals of therapy, and criteria for response.

HISTORY

Chemotherapy dates back to the early Greeks and Egyptians, who used metallic salts made from arsenic, copper, and lead. By the late 1800s, potassium arsenite and antimicrobials were used effectively to treat disease. In the early 1940s, hormonal therapies for breast and prostate cancers became available. World War II, however, is considered the true dawning of chemotherapy; researchers advanced the effectiveness of poisonous gas, nutrition, and antibiotics as viable cancer therapies.

Drug development increased with the establishment of the National Cancer Institute in 1953. For several decades, chemotherapy has cured a high proportion of patients with Hodgkin's disease, non-Hodgkin's lymphoma, testicular cancer, and acute lymphocytic leukemia of childhood. Chemotherapy used in conjunction with other cancer treatments has resulted in improved morbidity and mortality statistics in cancers of the breast, small-cell lung cancer, and osteosarcoma.

VOCABULARY

A glossary at the end of this book provides a vocabulary of cancer treatments and aspects of chemotherapy. However, the following words and phrases are worth highlighting now:

- Tumor: A collection of cancer cells. A tumor can be benign or malignant.
- Malignant: Growth that is not controlled, can invade through adjacent tissues, and can spread throughout the body.
- Benign: Abnormal growth that is not malignant.
- Cytotoxic agents, antineoplastic agents: Drugs used to kill cells.
- Neoplasm: Cancer or malignant cells.
- Metastasize: To spread to neighboring or distant organs or tissues.
- Proliferate: To grow or increase rapidly.
- Solid tumor: Cancers not classified as hematologic malignancies.

EFFECTIVENESS OF CHEMOTHERAPY

Chemotherapeutic agents are used systemically to treat cancers such as leukemias, lymphomas, and solid tumors. They also are used to treat undetectable metastases or to reduce the size or number of metastases. Table 1-1 lists types of cancer that respond to chemotherapy. Chemotherapy alone is the treatment of choice in hematologic malignancies, such as leukemia or lymphatic tumors, that have no localized focus of disease. Moreover, chemotherapy has been successful in the treatment of certain lymphomas and leukemias, allowing patients complete or partial remissions. Thousands of children with acute lymphocytic leukemia, who even 15 years ago would not have survived a year past diagnosis, have now reached adulthood disease-free because of advances in chemotherapy.

Adjuvant chemotherapy is one advance in the treatment of cancer. Courses of chemotherapy are used after surgery or radiation treatment of the primary lesion in an attempt to destroy any remaining cancer cells and to prevent local or metastatic recurrent disease. Adjuvant chemotherapy may be recommended even when patients have no clinical evidence of disease.

In general, most cancer chemotherapy regimens combine different drugs. Combination therapies have gained popularity and effectiveness since the late 1960s. Two or more drugs given together are more effective than one agent given alone. Combination therapy can lessen the cumulative toxic side effects of treatment and can allow specific separate drugs to be given at higher doses. Combination chemotherapy also can provide a synergy of action against cancer cell growth and proliferation and can delay the occurrence of drug resistance to specific agents. Chapter 7 provides some common combination chemotherapeutic regimens.

Although numerous factors determine the success of any choice of treatment, certain types of cancer are more sensitive to and respond more favorably to chemotherapy than others (Table 1-1). The degree of tumor sensitivity can be one of the important determinants in establishing a treatment plan and in predicting treatment outcome (Burnett, 1982).

Table 1-1

Classification of Tumors According to General Sensitivity to Chemotherapy

I. Cancers responding to chemotherapy; some percentage of patients will achieve long-term disease-free survival and most others will experience prolonged survival

Burkitts lymphoma	Choriocarcinoma
Acute lymphocytic leukemia in children	Acute myelogenous leukemia
Embryonal rhabdomyosarcoma	Ewing sarcoma
Hodgkin's disease	Non-Hodgkin's lymphomas
Testicular carcinoma	Wilms tumor
Lymphocytic lymphoma	Multiple myeloma

II. Advanced cancers responding to chemotherapy or hormonal therapy; chemotherapy commonly results in prolongation of survival

Adrenal cortical carcinoma	Breast carcinoma
Chronic myelogenous leukemia	Chronic lymphocytic leukemia
Ovarian carcinoma	Prostatic carcinoma
Small-cell carcinoma of the lung	Soft-tissue sarcoma
Squamous carcinoma of the head and neck	

III. Advanced cancers marginally responsive or unresponsive to chemotherapy

Colon carcinoma	Endometrial carcinoma
Gastric carcinoma	Glioblastoma
Bladder cancer	Carcinoma of the cervix
Central nervous system cancers	Hypernephroma
Epidermoid carcinoma of the lung	Esophageal carcinoma
Malignant carcinoid tumors	Hepatocellular carcinoma
Pancreatic carcinoma	Carcinoma of the penis
Thyroid carcinoma	

Adapted by Ellen Carr, RN, MSN

GOALS OF CHEMOTHERAPY

Although ridding a patient of the malignancy is the obvious intent of chemotherapy, that goal is not always achievable. Therefore, a review of the goals of cancer treatment is important.

Cure

Persons who have cancer are considered cured when they have remained free of cancer and have the same life expectancy as persons who do not have cancer. Five- and 10-year survival rates after treatment are benchmarks in establishing that a cure has occurred. Cure via chemotherapy occurs most often in patients who have highly proliferative cancers, such as acute lymphocytic leukemia, Hodgkins disease, or neuroblastoma in children. (See Chapter 2 for a more detailed explanation of chemotherapy effect on these cancers.) Generally, advanced solid tumors are not curable by chemotherapy. Notable exceptions are metastatic testicular cancer and gestational trophoblastic neoplasms (Samson, M. K.; Revkin, S. E.; Jones, S. E., 1984).

Control

Often when disease recurs after primary treatment or if metastases develop, cure is generally not possible. The goal of therapy then becomes to prolong survival and minimize symptoms. In some cases, chemotherapy can control metastatic disease and allow patients to maintain their quality of life for many months or even years, depending on the type and extent of the cancer. Malignancies that can be controlled by chemotherapy include breast cancer, Ewing sarcoma, prostatic cancer, multiple myeloma, and small-cell cancer of the lung.

Palliation

Palliative treatment lessens the patient's symptoms but does not cure the underlying disease. Once the cancer does not respond to available therapy, and a remission of the disease is no longer feasible, chemotherapy can be used to alleviate the symptoms of advanced disease. For example, drugs can be used to treat the complications of metastatic disease, such as hypercalcemia or pain (originating from pressure on nerves, lymphatics, the vascular system, or obstructed organs).

TUMOR RESPONSE CRITERIA

Standardized criteria have been established to assess treatment effectiveness. Criteria include survival rates, degree of response or remission, and duration of response.

- Complete response or remission (CR): The complete disappearance of all evidence of disease for more than one month.
- Partial response (PR): A reduction in measurable tumor mass of 50% or more of the original size for at least one month. Moreover, no evidence of new disease is seen, and the patient shows subjective improvement.
- Stable disease (SD): Tumor regression of 25% or less with or without subjective improvement.
- Progression: Clinical evidence of advancing disease during chemotherapy. This may include new tumor growth, new metastases, or reappearance of old lesions. If an adequate trial of therapy has been conducted, progression of the disease indicates a treatment failure.

Because improved quality of life is an important goal of cancer treatment, the benefits of chemotherapy should outweigh the detrimental side effects. Therefore, the ultimate goal of chemotherapy always is to enable a patient to stay active and/or feel better.

EXAM QUESTIONS

Chapter 1

Questions 1–5

1. What are primary goals of chemotherapy?

    a. Cure or control the growth of tumors to minimize symptoms
    b. Control tumor growth and boost immune system
    c. Expose cancer and relieve symptoms
    d. Stimulate tumor growth and boost immune system

2. Under what circumstances is a person who has cancer considered cured?

    a. The person has recurrence of disease eight years after treatment.
    b. The person remains disease-free and has a life expectancy five years shorter than a person without cancer.
    c. The person has recurrence of disease five years after treatment.
    d. The person remains disease-free and has the same life expectancy as a person without cancer.

3. Which of the following types of cancer is most sensitive to chemotherapy?

    a. Esophageal carcinoma
    b. Malignant melanoma
    c. Leukemias in children
    d. Hypernephroma

4. Stable disease (SD) refers to a measurable regression of tumor mass of what percentage with or without subjective improvement?

    a. 15% or less
    b. 25% or less
    c. 50% or more
    d. 75% or more

5. A partial response to treatment is a reduction in tumor size of at least

    a. 50%
    b. 25%
    c. 75%
    d. 90%

CHAPTER 2

BIOLOGY OF CHEMOTHERAPY

CHAPTER OBJECTIVE

After completing this chapter, you will be able to discuss the phases of the cell cycle and why chemotherapy can affect or destroy cancer cells.

LEARNING OBJECTIVES

After reading this chapter, you will be able to

1. Explain the phases of the cell cycle and what happens during each phase.
2. Describe theories such as the growth fraction that explain how cell numbers increase or remain constant.
3. Indicate how tumor cell kill can be orchestrated and what factors might interfere with that strategy.

Cellular kinetics (how cells grow and divide) are interrupted by chemotherapy during cancer treatment. As related to cancer cells, cellular kinetics discussed here mean the cell cycle, the division rate of cells (proliferation and growth fraction), and the cell kill theory.

CELL CYCLE

As Figure 2-1 shows, all human cells (normal and malignant) go through four phases in their growth: G_1, S, G_2, and M. A cell also can go into a fifth or resting stage, the G_0 phase. (Sometimes this resting stage is labeled as a separate phase or as part of the beginning of the G_1 phase.) No matter what the resting stage of a cell is called, the major action stages of cell growth are G_1, S, G_2, and M. Cells can remain in phases for an extended time period, but, in general, the cell cycle is one to five days.

During G_1, proteins and ribonucleic acid (RNA) are synthesized. A cell can stay in this stage for 8 to 48 hours. This is the most variable time of all the phases. If many cells are in G_1, the tumor will grow more slowly. If few cells are in G_1, the tumor grows more rapidly. This first stage, G_1, is preparation for S, the period when synthesis of deoxyribonucleic acid (DNA) takes place. During phase S, a period of 10 to 30 hours, chromosomes double. After S, a second G phase begins, when more RNA and protein synthesis occurs. This second growth phase of a few hours, called G_2, also begins the formation of spindle of chromosomes so that the cell is ready to divide. After G_2, the cell progresses to the M phase, or mitosis. The cell divides now in about an hour. In M, the parent cell divides into two daughter cells; all the genetic material is distributed evenly between the two daughters. These new daughter cells enter a resting

Figure 2-1
Cell Generation Cycle

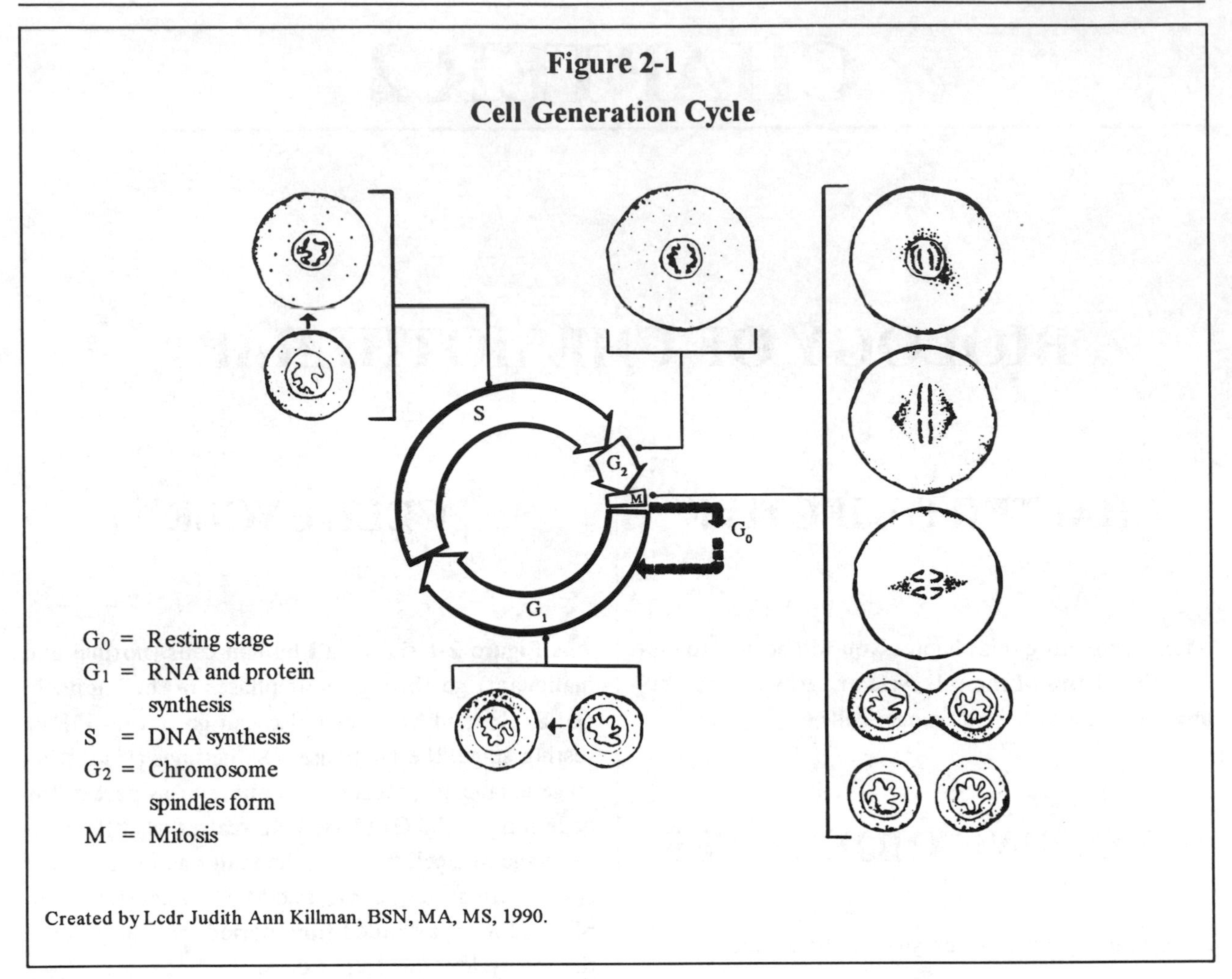

Created by Lcdr Judith Ann Killman, BSN, MA, MS, 1990.

phase (the G_0 phase) or enter G_1 to start the progression of the cell cycle all over again.

The period of G_1 through M is called the cell's generation time. This period can last hours or years, depending on the cell. When cells are exposed to chemotherapeutic agents, the generation time can change, thus interfering with stages of the cell cycle. The cycle is either altered or stopped entirely. Moreover, chemotherapeutic agents can affect cells at only certain phases in their cell cycles. Tables 2-1 and 2-2 indicate which agents are cell-cycle specific and which are not. Oncologists choose agents that are cell-cycle-phase specific, cell-cycle-phase nonspecific, or a combination of the two types. In general, the cell cycle of a tumor (one mitosis to the next mitosis) is one to five days.

GROWTH RATE OF CELLS

Cancer cells develop and mature just as normal cells do. Unfortunately, cancer cells bypass the biological feedback controls that would stop their aberrant growth or proliferation.

When administration of chemotherapy is considered in terms of the proliferation and growth fraction are key concepts. Oncologists apply these concepts when they choose chemotherapeutic agents, doses, and schedules that will result in killing the most cancer cells.

Cancer cells are more sensitive to chemotherapeutic agents when the cells are proliferating (in the pro-

Table 2-1
Cell-Cycle-Phase Specific Agents

G_1 Phase
Asparaginase
Prednisone

S Phase
Cytarabine
5-Fluorouracil
Hydroxyurea
Methotrexate
Thioguanine
Fludarabine
Clodribine
Mercaptopurine
Pentostatin

G_2 Phase
Bleomycin
Teniposide
Etoposide

Mitosis
Vinblastine
Vincristine
Vindesine
Paclitaxel
Vinorelbine

Table 2-2
Cell-Cycle-Phase Nonspecific Agents

Alkylating Agents
Busulfan
Chlorambucil
Ifosfamide
Carboplatin
Cisplatin
Cyclophosphamide
Mechlorethamine
Melphalan

Antibiotics
Dactinomycin
Daunorubicin
Doxorubicin
Idarubicin
Mitomycin

Nitrosoureas
Carmustine (BCNU)
Lomustine (CCNU)
Streptozocin

Miscellaneous
Dacarbazine
Procarbazine

Created by Lcdr Judith Ann Killman, BSN, MA, MS, 1990.

Figure 2-2

Action of Antineoplastic Agents in Relation to the Cell Cycle

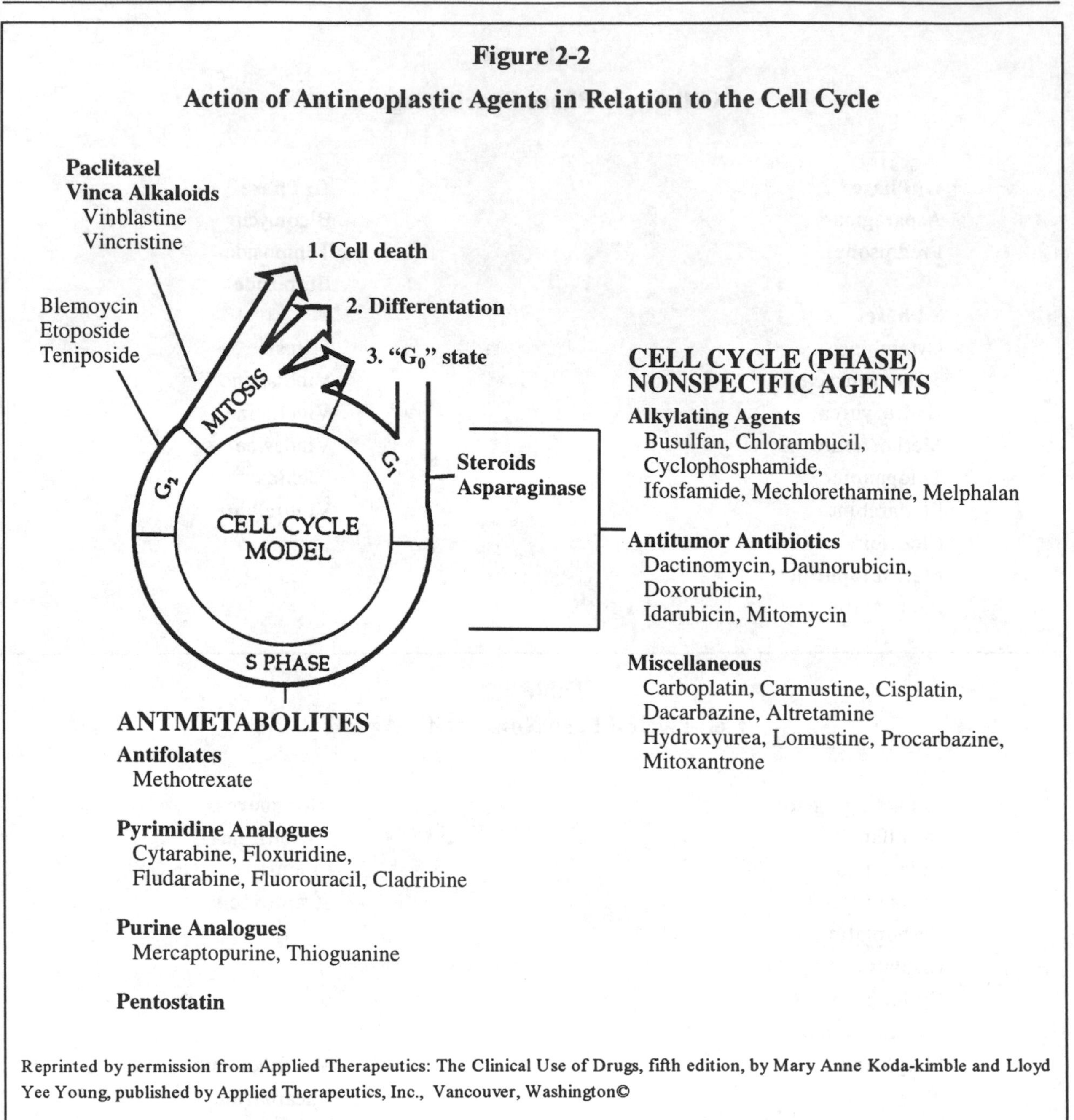

Reprinted by permission from Applied Therapeutics: The Clinical Use of Drugs, fifth edition, by Mary Anne Koda-kimble and Lloyd Yee Young, published by Applied Therapeutics, Inc., Vancouver, Washington©

gress of dividing). Cells that are dividing rapidly are most sensitive to chemotherapy. Some agents target just this phase of the cell cycle while others may affect the cell during any phase. Figure 2-2 shows chemotherapeutic agents and the phase of the cycle in which they are active.

Also, chemotherapy is more effective when a tumor is small (fewer cancer cells) and localized (no metastases). Therefore, the size of the tumor and the extent of its spread are crucial elements in cancer treatment. In some cases, chemotherapeutic agents might not be administered until the tumor has been reduced by surgery or irradiation. Alternatively, certain drugs are given first to reduce the size of a tumor, and then other drugs are targeted toward the smaller tumor mass.

The growth fraction is the ratio of the actively dividing cell population to the total cell population. Early-stage, small tumors have a high growth fraction and rapid tumor doubling time. Thus, small tumors grow more rapidly than larger tumors, and this may explain why chemotherapy is more effective against small tumors. (The tumor doubling time is the average length of time that cells need to reproduce themselves.)

Chemotherapy is used during the time when the cell population is dividing as part of a strategy to optimize cell death during this rapid period of tumor growth. Therefore, chemotherapy is most effective when tumor cells are rapidly dividing. As tumor burden increases, the doubling time is much longer, creating a plateau in the growth of the tumor and decreasing the effectiveness of chemotherapy.

The theory behind tumor growth can, in part, be explained on the basis of the Gompertzian model or function (see Figure 2-3). The model shows that early, small tumors grow rapidly. Then, as tumor bulk increases, the doubling time slows. (A larger tumor needs more blood and nutrients to sustain itself. If those supplies are diminished, the tumor cannot grow as rapidly.)

CELL KILL HYPOTHESIS

According to the most prominent cell kill theory, a percentage of the total number of cancer cells in the tumor will be killed with each course of chemotherapy. This theory is the rationale for using repeated doses of chemotherapeutic agents to reduce the total cell number. For example, an agent is intended to kill 90% of the cancer cells during the first course of treatment. During the second course, the remaining 10% of cancer cells are bombarded with the agent in hopes of reducing that 10% by another 90%. If a tumor has 1,000,000 cells to start, the first course will reduce the number of cells to 100,000. The second course will reduce the number of cells to 10,000, and so on.

The equations of this hypothesis do not include the number of cancer cells added to the tumor mass between the two courses of treatment if the chemotherapy is not working. Chemotherapy may be ineffective because cancer cells can remain or grow between courses if the scheduling of the agents is less than optimal, the growth fraction of the tumor is greater than the agent can control, or the cells are resistant to the lethal effects of the chemotherapy.

According to cell kill theory, if chemotherapy is working, then only a few cancer cells might remain after several courses of treatment. The person's immune system, according to this theory, may kill the remaining minimal number of cells (see Figure 2-4). Therefore, the cell kill theory makes sense under the following conditions:

1. All cells in a tumor population are equally sensitive to chemotherapy.

2. Cells do not change in their degree of responsiveness to chemotherapy over time.

3. Cells do not re-grow between course of therapy.

Despite the theories behind chemotherapy destroying cancer cells, some cancer cells die spontaneously because of decreased nutrition, genetic damage, or an unexpected inability to divide. Thus the cell kill theory can never be justified entirely. Unfortunately for many patients with various types of cancer, increases in tumor volume occur (called a recurrence or progression). Therefore, more explanations for tumor biology are needed so that strategies for giving chemotherapy can be optimized.

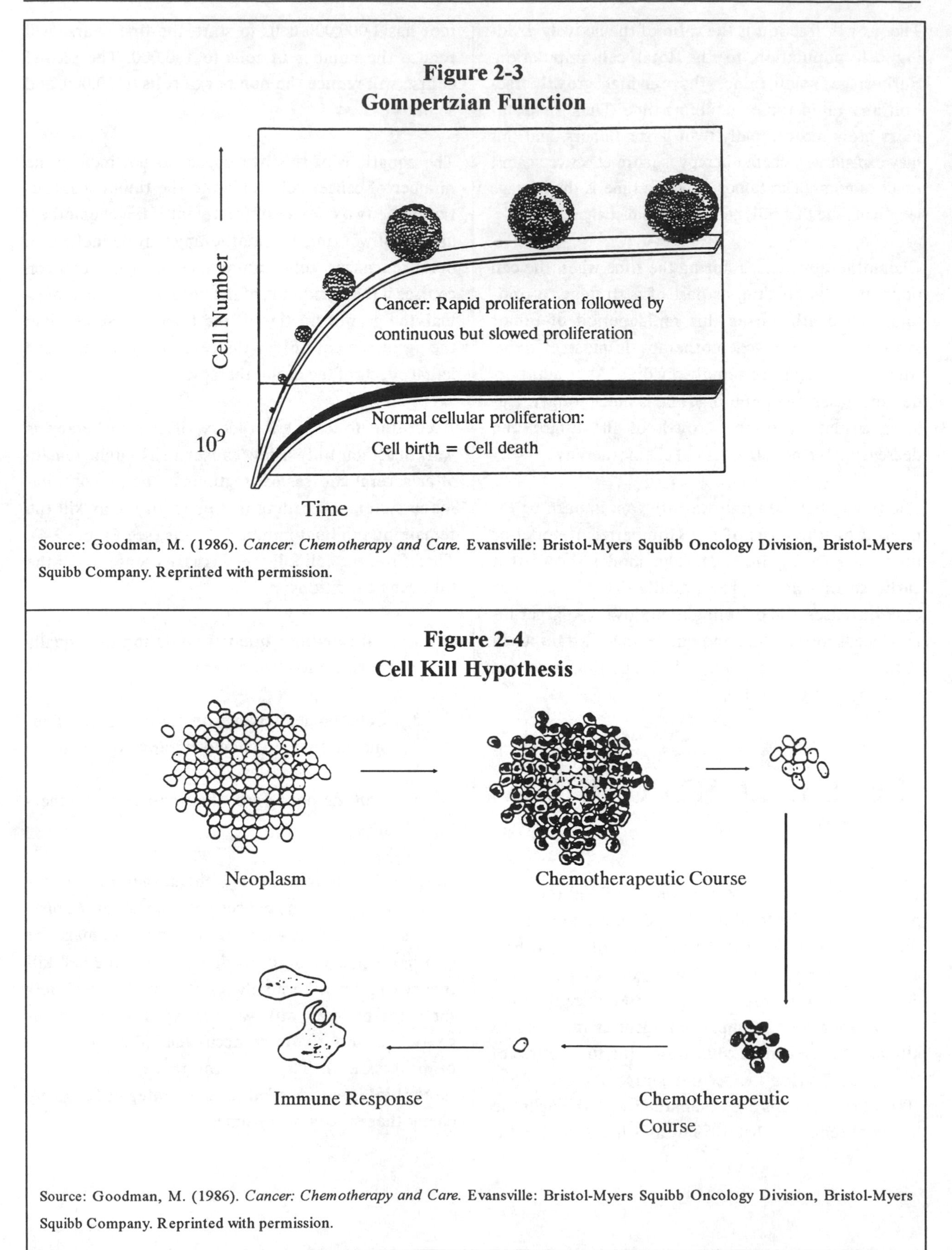

Figure 2-3
Gompertzian Function

Source: Goodman, M. (1986). *Cancer: Chemotherapy and Care.* Evansville: Bristol-Myers Squibb Oncology Division, Bristol-Myers Squibb Company. Reprinted with permission.

Figure 2-4
Cell Kill Hypothesis

Source: Goodman, M. (1986). *Cancer: Chemotherapy and Care.* Evansville: Bristol-Myers Squibb Oncology Division, Bristol-Myers Squibb Company. Reprinted with permission.

EXAM QUESTIONS

Chapter 2

Questions 6–10

6. What is the first phase of the cell cycle?

   a. G_1
   b. G_2
   c. Mitosis
   d. S

7. The response to chemotherapy is better when the tumor cells are doing which of the following?

   a. Resting
   b. Dividing rapidly
   c. Dividing slowly
   d. Changing their appearance

8. Which of the following drugs act on all phases of the cell cycle?

   a. Vinblastine, procarbazine, 5FU
   b. Cisplatin, BCNU, doxorubicin
   c. Prednisone, methotrexate, CCNU
   d. Bleomycin, vincristine, busulfan

9. The tumor growth fraction is the ratio of the actively dividing cell population to the number of

   a. Total cell population
   b. Cells without oxygen
   c. Cells with oxygen
   d. Cells going through one phase of the cell cycle

10. According to the cell kill hypothesis, an agent kills approximately what percentage of cancer cells?

    a. 10%
    b. 90%
    c. 75%
    d. 40%

CHAPTER 3

DRUG CLASSIFICATIONS

CHAPTER OBJECTIVE

After completing this chapter, you will be able to discuss classifications of chemotherapeutic agents and how these agents act on malignant and normal cells.

LEARNING OBJECTIVES

After reading this chapter, for various categories of chemotherapeutic agents, you will be able to

1. Identify their mechanism of action on a cancer cell.
2. Indicate common side effects of agents in the category.
3. Choose an agent (generic and trade name) that is represented by that catcgory.

Many chemotherapeutic agents are available to treat malignancies. Chapter 5 highlights a few of the more common agents. This chapter focuses on classifications of those agents. Despite their similar modes of action, various agents within a class may be active against different tumor types. Agents within a class may also share some common toxicites (e.g., bone marrow suppression) as well as produce unique adverse effects. The mechanism of action, disease sensitivity and toxicity profile are all considered when selecting a chemotherapeutic agent.

The seven categories of chemotherapeutic agents described here are all represented in Chapter 5. The categories are alkylating agents, antimetabolites, antitumor antibiotics, nitrosoureas, plant alkaloids, hormones, and a miscellaneous group. Table 3-1 gives a partial list of classifications and specific drugs. (Note: In the narrative of this curriculum, the generic names of a drug are listed first and then the trade or manufacturer's name in parentheses ( ) and other synonyms in brackets [ ]).

ALKYLATING AGENTS

Alkylating agents are one of the more commonly prescribed classes of chemotherapeutic agents. This class also is said to be the first recognized type of chemotherapeutic agent. Mecholrethamine or nitrogen mustard, the first effective chemotherapeutic agent, is a derivative of a chemical warfare gas. Its effectiveness as a therapy for Hodgkin's disease was first recognized in 1945 after World War II. Now, other less toxic alkylating agents are more often used. Nevertheless, mecholrethomine is the prototype with which all subsequent alkylating agents are compared.

Table 3-1

Chemotherapeutic Agents According to Classification

Generic Name (Tradename) [Other Synonyms]

Alkylating Agents (Classic)
Busulfan (Myleran®)
Chlorambucil (Leukeran®)
Cyclophosphamide (Cytoxan®)
Ifosfamide (Ifex®) (Isophosphamide)
Mechlorethamine (Mustargen®) [Nitrogen mustard]
Melphalan (Alkeran®)

Antitumor Antibiotics
Bleomycin (Blenoxane®)
Dactinomycin (Cosmegan®) [Actinomycin D]
Daunorubicin (Cerubidine®) [Daunomycin]
Doxorubicin (Adriamycin®)
Idarubicin (Indamycin®)
Mitomycin (Mutamycin®) [Mitomycin C]
Plicamycin (Mithracin®) [Mithramycin]
Procarbazine (Matulane®)

Other Alkylating-Like Agents
Carboplatin (Paraplatin®) [CBDCA]
Carmustine (BiCNU®) [BCNU]
Cisplatin (Platinol®) [Cisplatinum, DDP]
Lomustine (CeeNu®) [CCNU]
Mitoxantrone (Novantrone®) [DHAD, dihydroxyanthracenedione]
Streptozocin (Zanosar®)
Thiotepa [triethylenethiophosphoramide]

Antimetabolites
Cladribine (Leustatin®) [2-CDA]
Cytarabine (Cytosar-U®) [Ara-C]
Floxuridine (FUDR®)
Fludarabine (Fludara®)
Fluorouracil [5-FU, 5-fluorouracil]
Hydroxyurea (Hydrea®)
Mercaptopurine [6-MP, 6-mercaptopurine]
Methotrexate (Mexate®) [MTX]
Pentostatin (Nipent®) [2'-Deoxycoformycin]
Thioguanine [6-TG, 6-thioguaine]

Plant Alkaloids
Etoposide (Vepesid®) [VP-16, VP-16-213]
Paclitaxel (Taxol®)
Teniposide (Vumon®) [VM-26]
Vinblastine (Velban®)
Vincristine (Oncovin®)
Vinorelbine (Navelbine®)

Miscellaneous
Altretamine (Hexalen®) [hexamethylmelamine]
Asparaginase (Elspar®)
Pegaspargase (Oncaspar®) [PEG-L-asparaginase]
Mitotane (Lysodren®) [*o,p'*-DDD]

Created by Ellen Carr, RN, MSN, and Lcdr Judith Ann Killman, BSN, MA, MS, 1990. Revised by Rebecca S. Finley, PharmD, MS

Alkylating agents can affect all phases of the cell cycle. Their mechanism of action is called alkylation. The drug binds with DNA, often causing breaks and preventing DNA replication. Because DNA is essential for life and growth, alkylating agents can stop tumor cells from growing and dividing. Most alkylating agents are cell-cycle phase nonspecific, but rapidly dividing cells are most sensitive to alkylation.

Alkylating agents, like all chemotherapeutic agents, affect both normal and tumor cells. These agents affect the most rapidly proliferating cells, namely, those in the bone marrow, the gastrointestinal (GI) tract, the hair follicles, and the gonads.

Examples of alkylating agents are cyclophosphamide (Cytoxan®), busulfan (Myleran®), and mechlorethamine (Mustargen®).

ANTIMETABOLITES

Antimetabolites inactivate enzymes or alter the structure of DNA, thereby changing the DNA's ability to replicate. Because antimetabolites can substitute for the nucleotides that form the DNA's helix, aberrant molecules can form. These molecules stop the cell's ability to develop or replicate.

Antimetabolites are drugs that are structurally similar to the nucleotides: cytosine, thymine, adenine, and guanine. They act in three ways:

1. Substitution: The drug takes the place of a natural metabolite, thereby altering the function of the molecule.

2. Competition: The drug occupies an enzyme-binding site, thereby preventing the normal compound from binding.

3. Noncompetitive binding or irreversible binding: The drug occupies enzyme-binding sites and inactivates those sites.

Because antimetabolites interfere with DNA synthesis, many of them are S-phase specific. They are most effective against tumors that have a high growth fraction (rapidly growing tumors).

Common side effects of antimetabolites are bone marrow suppression and toxic effects to cells in the GI tract.

Examples of antimetabolites are methotrexate [MTX], a folate antagonist; 6-mercaptopurine [6MP], a purine antagonist; fluorouracil [5FU], a pyrimidine antagonist; and cytarabine [Cytosar-U®, ARA-C] a cytidine antagonist.

ANTITUMOR ANTIBIOTICS

Antitumor antibiotics are the fermentation products of microorganisms. They have anti-infective properties but are not used to fight infections. They are cytotoxic. Their actions are similar to those of alkylating agents. They bind to DNA so that DNA and RNA transcription is blocked.

The half-life of some of these drugs is several days, so their side effects can be slow to diminish. Some antitumor antibiotics can still be cytotoxic after they have been metabolized by the liver.

Side effects can be similar to those of alkylating agents, namely bone marrow suppression and GI toxic effects. Extravasation and tumor necrosis also may occur. Moreover, some antitumor antibiotics can be toxic to cardiac or pulmonary tissue. These drugs are active in all phases of the cell cycle.

Examples of antitumor antibiotics are daunorubicin hydrochloride (Cerubidine®), plicamycin (Mithracin), doxorubicin hydrochloride (Adriamycin®), and bleomycin sulfate (Blenoxane®).

PLANT ALKALOIDS

Vinca alkaloids act as "spindle poisons." During the metaphase (M) of mitosis, the mitotic spindles attach to the strands of DNA, pulling the strands to each end of the cell so that the strands can divide. Vinca alkaloids bind to the microtubules of the spindles causing mitosis to stop. Thus, these drugs are cell-cycle phase specific.

The name vinca alkaloids comes from *Vinca rosea,* the periwinkle plant from which they are made. Examples of vinca alkaloids are vinblastine sulfate (Velban) and vincristine sulfate (Oncovin). Vinca alkaloids can be toxic to bone marrow and peripheral nerves. They can also cause severe tissue damage if extravasated.

Etoposide [VP16] and teniposide [VM-26] are derivatives of *Podophyllum pellatum*, the May apple. They are active in late S phase, in G_2, and in mitosis. Etoposide can trigger severe hypotension, especially if administered too rapidly.

NITROSOUREAS

Nitrosoureas sometimes are categorized with alkylating agents because they act like alkylating agents by interfering with DNA replication and RNA synthesis. They are cell-cycle-phase nonspecific. Because they are lipid soluble, they can cross the blood-brain barrier. Therefore, they can be used to treat brain or central nervous system (CNS) malignancies. They can be toxic to GI and bone marrow cells. These drugs have a prolonged effect on the bone marrow, so they are not given as frequently as other drugs. The toxic effects can be controlled somewhat when dose limits are imposed.

Examples of nitrosoureas are carmustine, streptozocin, and lomustine.

HORMONES

Hormones used to treat cancer interfere with protein synthesis and change cell metabolism by altering the hormonal environment of the cell. They attempt to turn off the tumor growth in tissues dependent on hormones; such tissues include the breast, prostate, and endometrium. Hormonal therapies, in general, are not used to produce a cure but to provide control and palliation. Toxic effects can be minor and well tolerated. Categories of hormone therapies (with examples of specific drugs in parentheses) are antiestrogens (tamoxifen), androgens (testosterone), corticosteroids (prednisone, hydrocortisone), estrogens (estradiol), and progestins (Megace®, Provera®).

MISCELLANEOUS AGENTS

The general category of miscellaneous agents includes metals such as cisplatin (Platinol®). Cisplatin inhibits DNA, protein, and RNA synthesis. Cisplatin is cell-cycle-phase nonspecific. It can be toxic to the GI tract, otic nerves, and the kidneys. Carboplatin, a close derivative of cisplatin, is less toxic to inner ear and kidney cells but more toxic to the bone marrow.

L-asparaginase is an enzyme that inhibits protein synthesis by depriving cells of required amino acids, thus blocking proliferation. The drug can cause allergic reactions and can be toxic to cells in the GI tract.

Chapter 5 describes other agents that do not fit into the standard categories of chemotherapeutic agents.

EXAM QUESTIONS

Chapter 3

Questions 11–15

11. What kind of tissues are affected most by alkylating agents?

    a. Slowly proliferating tissues
    b. Rapidly proliferating tissues
    c. Tissues located only in the pleural cavity
    d. Tissues located only in the brain

12. Two examples of alkylating agents are

    a. Cytoxan® and mechlorethamine
    b. Bleomycin and vinblastine
    c. Oncovin® and etoposide
    d. 5FU and carmustine

13. One example of a miscellaneous chemotherapeutic agent (not included in a standard category) is:

    a. Nitrogen mustard
    b. Cisplatin
    c. Methotrexate
    d. Vinblastine

14. Nitrosoureas have a mechanism of action like that of what other chemotherapeutic agents?

    a. Alkylating agents
    b. Hormones
    c. Enzymes
    d. Antitumor antibiotics

15. Which of the following statements about alkylating agents is correct?

    a. They are cell-cycle nonspecific.
    b. They are the same as hormones.
    c. They are cell-cycle specific.
    d. They were not developed until 1980.

CHAPTER 4

ADMINISTRATION OF CHEMOTHERAPEUTIC AGENTS

CHAPTER OBJECTIVES

After completing this chapter, you will be able to describe principles of safe administration of chemotherapeutic agents.

LEARNING OBJECTIVES

After reading this chapter, you will be able to

1. Describe the information needed before a chemotherapeutic agent is administered.
2. Identify four routes of administration for chemotherapeutic agents.
3. Describe three aspects of the care of central venous catheters.
4. Identify four ways to ensure that chemotherapeutic agents are handled and administered safely.

Administration of chemotherapeutic agents should include an organized, systematic approach to nursing care to ensure skilled, safe therapy for patients. Although the nurse's responsibility for administration can vary, depending on the health care setting, the basic principles are universal.

Each workplace or institution has established policies and procedures for administration of chemotherapy that are based on licensing and accreditation requirements. These policies and procedures should remain the ultimate guide. This chapter reviews standard components of administation, with the intent that you and your institution have customized these principles for your ongoing practice.

KNOWLEDGE ABOUT THE PATIENT

Before administering chemotherapeutic agents, you need to have recent, thorough data on the patient who will be receiving the drugs. This information should include (but not be limited to) assessment of the patient, both ongoing and immediately before administration, and knowledge of the patient's physical, psychosocial, and cognitive status. The patient's disease process, as indicated by diagnostic and laboratory findings, is important. You also need to know the patient's medical history with regard to previous chemotherapy, specifically the agents administered (dose, side effects experienced, method and site of administration, problems noted). Once you have all this information, administration of the current drug(s) can proceed.

KNOWLEDGE AND SKILLS NEEDED TO ADMINISTER THE AGENTS

Principles of safe handling of chemotherapeutic agents are discussed later in this chapter. Keep in mind that you should be cognizant of those principles as you complete the preadministration checklist. Although those principles are crucial, especially with agents administered through the arterial or venous system, you should still adhere to principles of safe handling (no matter what the route) throughout the administration process.

The following is a suggested checklist for the administration of any cytotoxic agent (Tenenbaum, 1987).

1. Verify the medication and the dose.

2. Review the patient's allergy history and relevant data (e.g., complete blood cell count, other laboratory findings).

3. Review the patient's history of any previous chemotherapy and related medications.

4. Teach the patient about the immediate and delayed side effects of the medications being given.

5. Use proper procedure to identify the patient.

6. Identify yourself to the patient and the patient's family and answer any questions they may have.

7. Establish that the patient has been informed of the risks and side effects of treatment.

8. Inform the patient or the patient's significant other to report all adverse effects.

9. Administer antiemetics or other premedications as ordered (or get an order if none has been written).

10. When administering medication, observe the five "rights":

    - Right patient
    - Right drug
    - Right dose
    - Right route
    - Right time

11. Always chart medication promptly according to your agency's policy.

Some specifics of this checklist deserve more comment: pertinent laboratory data, calculation of doses, route and technique of administration, informed consent, safe handling of the drugs, and documentation. (Chapter 6 reviews patient management issues including side effects, Chapter 5 reviews specific agents, and Chapter 7 includes combination therapies.)

Pertinent Laboratory Data

Before a patient receives chemotherapy, laboratory data should indicate that such treatment will be appropriate and safe. Most often, these data are blood counts and urine tests to determine the status of the patient's bone marrow, other blood components, and liver and renal function. Giving agents when blood counts are too low can compromise the patient's ability to tolerate the drug or its side effects. One common example of laboratory data that affect administration of chemotherapy is a low white blood cell (WBC) count.

The WBC count is the total number of white blood cells. The granulocyte count is another subdivision of WBCs. Granulocytes are one of three types of leukocytes. (The others are lymphocytes and monocytes.) Granulocytes usually make up about 70% of all WBCs. Granulocytes have three different categories. Neutrophils (or polymorphonuclear leukocytes [PMNs]) destroy bacteria and are the first fighters of infection. They are present during early, acute phases of inflammation. Eosinophils destroy bacteria but are more involved in combating allergic reactions. Basophils are involved in fighting acute allergic systemic reactions. Granulocyte counts are a way to evaluate a person's ability to fight off infection. A more extensive discussion of the effects of chemotherapy on the bone marrow follows in Chapter 6.

If the patient has limited ability to fight off infection because the number of white cells is reduced, administering additional chemotherapeutic agents, which will further suppress the WBC, can increase the risk. The physician may decide to delay administration of the agent until the WBC count rises, choose a different agent not so toxic to bone marrow cells, or eliminate administration of the agent entirely.

Another example of important laboratory data is the patient's renal status, as shown by creatinine clearance, levels of blood urea nitrogen, and serum creatinine, or urine output. Some chemotherapeutic agents are particularly toxic to the kidney. In addition, many other chemotherapy drugs are excreted through the kidneys; and if kidney function is inadequate, toxic drug levels may accumulate. Therefore, adequate renal status is a necessary prerequisite for the safe administraiton of chemotherapeutic drugs, especially those that have a significant effect on re[illegible] cells.

Thus, the nurse's knowledge and understanding of laboratory data are pivotal to the safe administration of chemotherapeutic agents. Table 4-1 lists important laboratory data to be gathered (with normal values for comparison).

Calculation of Doses

The dose of a chemotherapeutic agent most often is calculated by using formulas for determining the patient's body surface area. Doses are expressed as milligrams per body surface area given in square meters (mg/m^2). Height and weight determine body surface area. Dosages also can be expressed as milligrams per kilogram of body weight (mg/kg). Dosages determined on the basis of body surface area are more accurate because they take into account the size of the patient—an especially important difference between adults and children. Figure 4-1 is a series of nomograms, charts or graphs that can be used to determine a patient's body surface area.

Route and Technique of Administration

Agents can be administered in many ways. Factors that influence the choice of a route include the following:

- The optimal effects of the agent, in terms of how it is administered: Is a continual therapeutic blood level necessary? Can the agent be absorbed through the GI tract or cross the blood-brain barrier?
- The patient's ability to tolerate the agent: Can the patient swallow? Is the patient unconscious?
- The agent's effects on cells in the GI tract: Is the agent highly emetic?

Table 4-1
Laboratory Values That May Be Altered by Antineoplastic Agents

	NORMAL RANGE*		
TEST	**Conventional Units**	**S.I. Units**	**ALTERATION**
Complete blood count (CBC):			
Total leukocytes	4,500-11,000/cu mm	5.5–10.0 x 10^9/L	Decreased with all except asparaginase, bleomycin, and mitotane. Mild with vincristine.
Myelocytes	0	0	
Band neutrophils (bands)	150-400/cu mm (3-5%)	150-400 x 10^6/L	
Segmented neutrophils (segs)	3,000-5,800/cu mm (54-62%)	3000-5800 x 10^6/L	
Lymphocytes	1,500-3,000/cu mm (25-33%)	1500-3000 x 10^6/L	
Monocytes	300-500/cu mm (3-7%)	300-500 x 10^6/L	
Eosinophils	50-250/cu mm (1-3%)	50-250 x 10^6/L	
Basophils	15-50/cu mm (0-0.75%)	15-50 x 10^6/L	
Platelets	150,000-300,000/cu mm	150,000-300,000 x 10^9/L	As above.
Reticulocytes	0.5-1.5% of erythrocytes	25-75 x 10^9/L	
Hemoglobin	Male: 14.0-18.0 gm/dl Female: 12.0-16.0 gm/dl	Male: 2.17-2.79 mmol/L Female: 1.86-2.48 mmol/L	Some decrease with same medications that cause leukopenia. Note: The client may be anemic secondary to the disease and/or chemotherapy.
Hematocrit	Male: 30-54 mg/dl Female: 37-47 mg/dl	Male: 0.40-0.54 Female: 0.37-0.47	
Coagulation tests:			
Prothrombin time (PT) (one stage)	12.0 -14.0 sec	12.0-14.0 sec	May be prolonged with plicamycin.

Table 4-1
Laboratory Values That May Be Altered by Antineoplastic Agents
(*Continued*)

TEST	NORMAL RANGE* Conventional Units	S.I. Units	ALTERATION
Partial thromboplastin time	20-35 sec	20-35 sec	
Glucose, carbohydrate metabolism:			
Amylase, serum	25-135 milliunits/ml	25-125 units/L	May be increased with asparaginase.
Glucose (fasting)	60-110 mg/dl	3.33-5.55 mmol/L	May be increased with asparaginase, streptozocin. May be decreased with aminoglutethimide, busulfan.
Hepatic function tests:†			
Aspartate	8-20 milliunits/ml (30°)	8-20 units/L (30 C.)	
aminotransferase (AST)‡	7-40 milliunits/ml (37°)	7-40 units/L (37 C.)	May increase with hepatotoxicity due to aminoglutethimide, amsacrine, carmustine, chlorambucil, cyclophosphamide, cytarabine, dacarbazine, etoposide, floxuridine, 5-fluorouracil, lomustine, mercaptopurine, methotrexate, mitomycin, plicamycin, teniposide, thioguanine. Note: Transient elevation of enzymes (AST, ALT) with asparaginase, dacarbazine, etoposide. Transient elevation of alkaline phosphatase with etoposide.
Alanine	8-20 milliunits/ml (30°)	8-20 units/L (30 C.)	
aminotransferase (ALT)§	5-35 milliunits/ml (37°)	5-35 units/L (37 C.)	
Alkaline phosphatase	20-90 milliunits/ml (30°)	20-90 units/L (30 C.)	
Bilirubin, serum			
Total	0.3-1.1 mg/dl	5.1-19 umol/L	
Direct	0.1-0.4 mg/dl	1.7-6.8 umol/L	
Indirect	0.2-0.7 mg/dl (total minus direct)	3.4-12 umol/L	
Lactate dehydrogenase	45-90 milliunits/ml (I.U.) (30°)	45-90 units/L (30 C.)	
(LDH)	100-190 milliunits/ml (37°)	100-190 milliunits/ml (37 C.)	

Table 4-1
Laboratory Values That May Be Altered by Antineoplastic Agents
(*Continued*)

TEST	NORMAL RANGE* Conventional Units	NORMAL RANGE* S.I. Units	ALTERATION
Renal Function Tests:†			
Blood urea nitrogen	10-20 mg/dl	7.1-14.3 mmol/L	Elevation in BUN, creatinine with renal impairment with asparaginase, cisplatin, cytarabine, hydroxyurea, methotrexate, mitomycin, plicamycin.
(BUN) — blood plasma or serum	11-23 mg/dl	53-106 *u*mol/L	
Creatinine, serum	0.6-1.2 mg/dl		
Creatinine clearance	Male: 110-150 ml/min Female: 105-132 ml/min	110-150 ml/min 105-132 ml/min	Creatinine clearance may be prolonged with renal impairment. Note: Cisplatin, high-dose methotrexate may be withheld if clearance is below 60 ml/minute.
Electrolytes			
Calcium	4.5-5.5 mEq/L 9.0-11.0 mg/dl	2.25-2.75 mmol/L	May be decreased with cisplatin, plicamycin, streptozocin. May be increased with androgens, antiestrogens, estrogens, corticosteroids. Decreased with plicamycin.
Magnesium	1.5-2.5 mEq/l 1.8-3.0 mg/dl	0.75-1.25 mmol/L	May be decreased with cisplatin.
Potassium, serum	3.5-5.0 mEq/L	3.5-5.0 mmol/L	May be increased with aminoglutethimide, busulfan. (Note: Also increases as a result of rapid tumor cell lysis.) May be decreased with cisplatin, corticosteroids, plicamycin.
Sodium, serum	136-145 mEq/L	136-145 mmol/L	May be increased with androgens, antiestrogens, corticosteroids, estrogens, progestins. May be decreased with aminoglutethimide, busulfan, cisplatin, cyclophosphamide, ifosfamide, vinblastine, vincristine, vindesine.

* Normal ranges from Rakel, R. E. (ed.): *Conn's Current Therapy 1988*. Philadelphia, W.B. Saunders Co., 1988.

†Note: Normal hepatic, bilary, and renal function are necessary for metabolism and elimination of some chemotherapeutic agents. Some medications may be withheld or require dose reduction with compormised function of these systems. Consult manufacturers' literature under "Warnings," "Precautions," or "Dosage" for this information.

‡Formerly known as serum glutamic oxaloacetic transaminase (SGOT).

§Formerly known as serum glutamic pyruvic transaminase (SGPT).

Source: Tenenbaum, L. (1989). *Cancer chemotherapy: A reference guide* (pp. 271-302). Philadelphia: Saunders. Reprinted with permission.

Figure 4-1
Nomograms

Body Surface of Adults

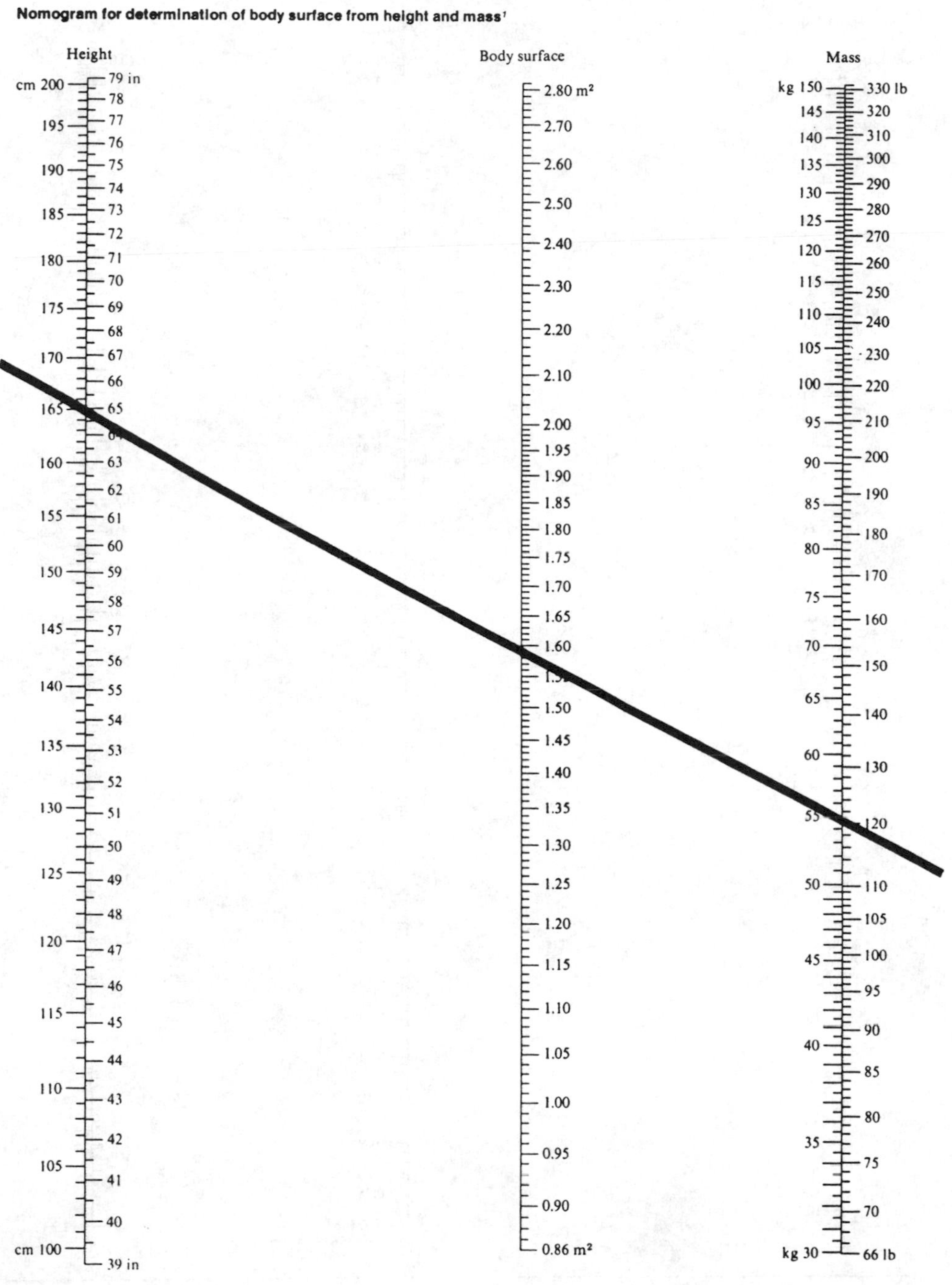

[1] From the formula of Du Bois and Du Bois, *Arch. intern. Med.*, 17, 863 (1916): $S = M^{0.425} \times H^{0.725} \times 71.84$, or $\log S = \log M \times 0.425 + \log H \times 0.725 + 1.8564$ (S: body surface in cm², M: mass in kg, H: height in cm).

Adult nomogram. (From C. Lentner (Ed.). (1981). *Geigy Scientific Tables*, (8th ed., vol. 1, p. 226). Basel: Ciba-Geigy. Reprinted with permission.)

Figure 4-1

Nomograms

Body Surface of Children

Nomogram for determination of body surface from height and mass[1]

Height — cm 120 – cm 25; 47 in – 10 in

Body surface — 1.10 m² – 0.074 m²

Mass — kg 40.0 – kg 1.0; 90 lb – 2.2 lb

[1] From the formula of DuBois and DuBois, *Arch. intern. Med.*, 17, 863 (1916): $S = M^{0.425} \times H^{0.725} \times 71.84$, or $\log S = \log M \times 0.425 + \log H \times 0.725 + 1.8564$ (S: body surface in cm², M: mass in kg, H: height in cm).

Pediatric nomogram used for calculation of the body surface area of a child, because the composition of a child's body differs somewhat from that of an adult. (From C. Lentner (Ed.). (1981). *Geigy Scientific Tables*, (8th ed., vol. 1, p. 227). Basel: Ciba-Geigy. Reprinted with permission.)

- The agent's effect on other tissues: Is the agent irritating to epithelial tissue?

Oral route. The oral route is chosen when the agent can be absorbed through the GI system.

Intramuscular and subcutaneous routes. The intramuscular (IM) and subcutaneous (SC) routes are used infrequently, and only with agents that are not vesicants. Use a small-gauge needle, be sure muscle or subcutaneous tissue at the site of administration is adequate, and cleanse the area with antiseptic solution. If the patient has thrombocytopenia (a decrease in the number of platelets), check for bleeding at the site of administration.

Intravenous route. The intravenous (IV) route is the most common route for administration of chemotherapeutic agents. Vesicants can be administered by this route. The following is a generic procedure for administering agents IV (Oncology Nursing Society, 1988).

1. Wash your hands (to prevent infection, phlebitis).
2. Prepare the skin per your institution's policy.
3. Use the smallest gauge needle possible with regard to vein size and objective of therapy.
4. Change the IV fluid every 24 hours and change tubing per your institution's policy.
5. Maintain aseptic technique in managing the IV system.
6. Check the IV insertion site and along the venous route for signs of infection: redness, warmth, pain, discharge, and odor.

Peripheral veins suitable for venipuncture should feel smooth and pliable, not hard or sclerotic. Select the site in an unhurried, methodical way (see Figure 4-2). The most appropriate site is the distal part of the arm. If repeated venipuncture is necessary and the other arm cannot be used, venipuncture should be done proximally to avoid leakage at the previous puncture site. Large veins in the forearm are preferred. If a drug does extravasate, soft tissue around those veins can limit functional impairment. Avoid the antecubital fossa and wrist if possible; extravasation in these areas can destroy nerves and tendons, affecting function.

Figure 4-2
Venipuncture Sites on the Arm

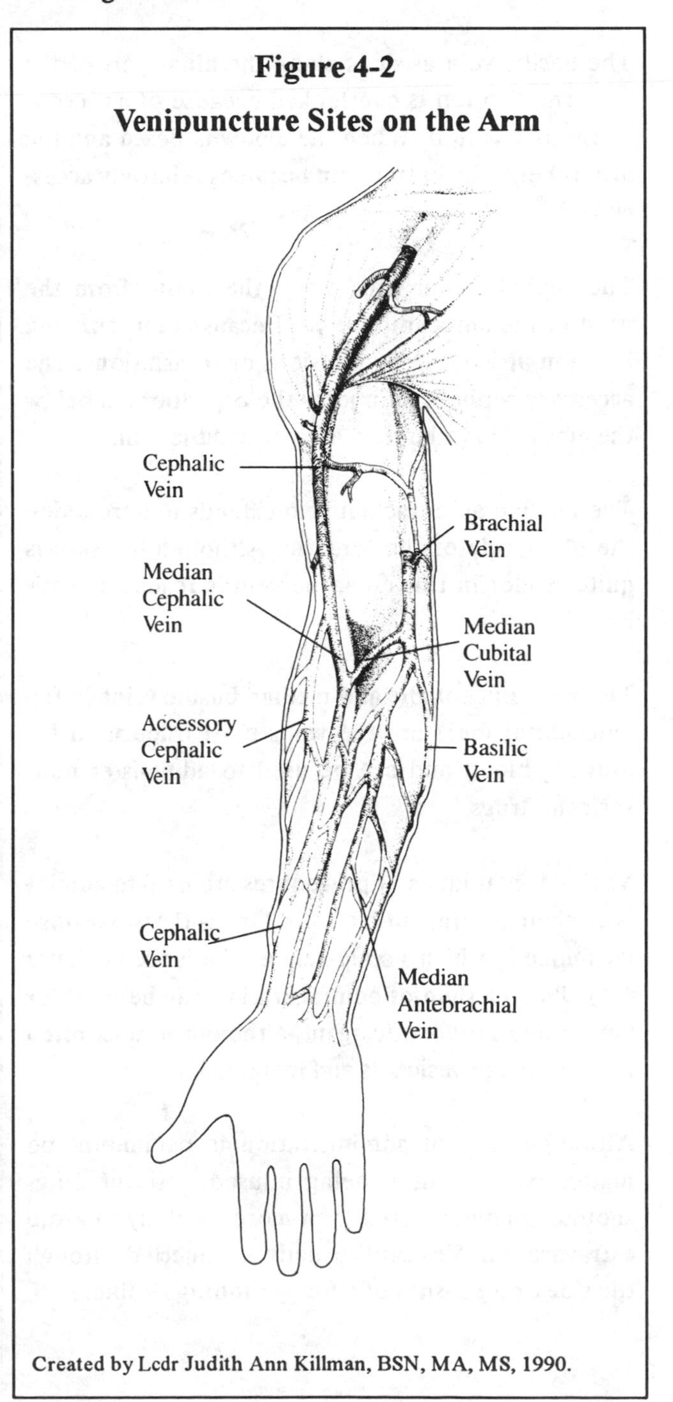

Created by Lcdr Judith Ann Killman, BSN, MA, MS, 1990.

The superficial veins of the upper extremities include the digital, metacarpal, cephalic, basilic, and median veins. The digital veins are not preferred sites for venipuncture, but with adequate stabilization they can be used for nonvesicants (see Figure 4-3). The metacarpal veins are formed by the union of the digital veins. Because of their location on the dorsum of the hand, they are relatively easy to stablize and enter with a scalp-vein needle or catheter.

The basilic vein ascends along the ulnar part of the forearm. It often is overlooked because of its inconspicuous location. When the elbow is flexed and the arm is bent, the basilic vein becomes relatively accessible.

The cephalic vein runs along the radius from the wrist to the antecubital fossa. Because of its size and location, it is ideal for infusions or transfusions. The accessory cephalic vein joins the cephalic vein below the elbow. It is a large, readily accessible vein.

The median antebrachial vein extends upward along the ulnar side of the forearm. Although the skin is quite tender in this area, the vein is readily accessible.

The median cephalic and median basilic veins in the antecubital fossa are the veins most often used for drawing blood and can be used to administer nonvesicant drugs.

Various techniques or procedures are used to administer chemotherapeutic agents. One is the two-syringe technique in which a scalp-vein needle is used (Figure 4-4). This method of administration can be used for any chemotherapeutic agent, although it most often is used for nonvesicants and irritants.

Although care in administration is paramount no matter what agent is being infused, vesicant drugs should be administered even more carefully to avoid extravasation. Vesicants usually are injected through the side arm (Y-site) of a freely running IV line.

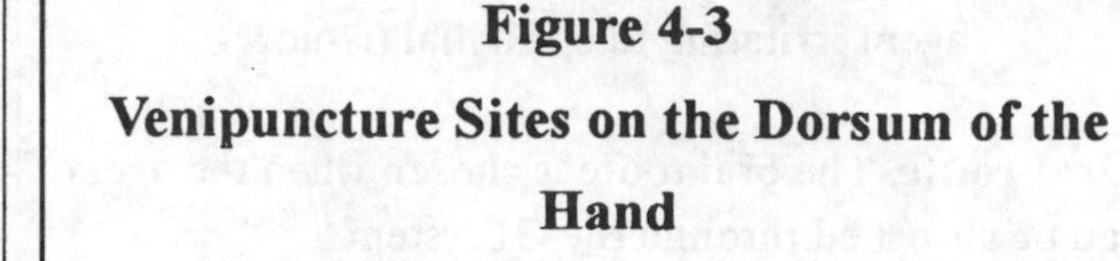

Figure 4-3

Venipuncture Sites on the Dorsum of the Hand

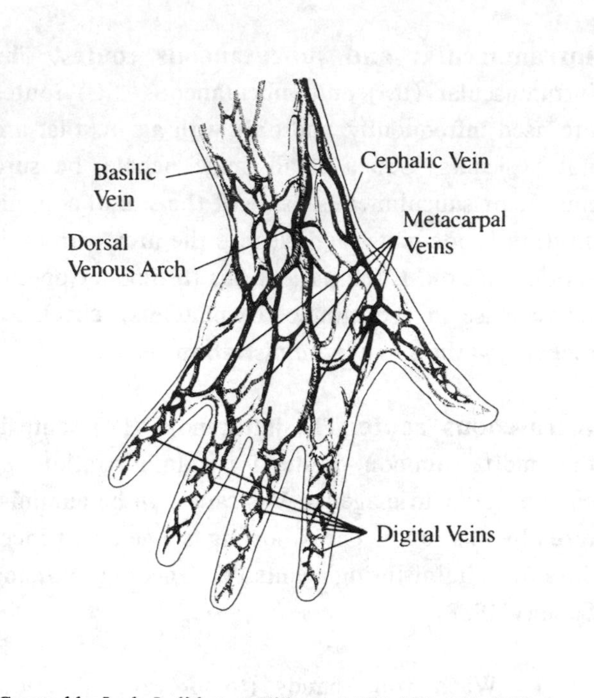

Created by Lcdr Judith Ann Killman, MSN, MA, MS, 1990.

Establish IV access with good blood return and a stable catheter site. Experts do not agree on the order in which vesicant drugs should be given when more than one agent is being administered. Some say the vesicant should be given first, others say it should be given last. Once again, refer to your own institution's policies as the main guide in your practice setting.

If a nonvesicant drug infiltrates during administration, stop the infusion and change sites. Continue to watch the site of infiltration and provide comfort measures as needed. Infiltration (extravasation) of vesicants is discussed in Chapter 6.

Venous access devices. IV drugs often are administered through peripheral veins. However, for patients who require continued IV access, use of a central venous access device (VAD) (also called central catheter) is an effective means for administration (see Table 4-2). (These catheters also can be used to

Figure 4-4
Venipuncture and Administration of Chemotherapeutic Drugs

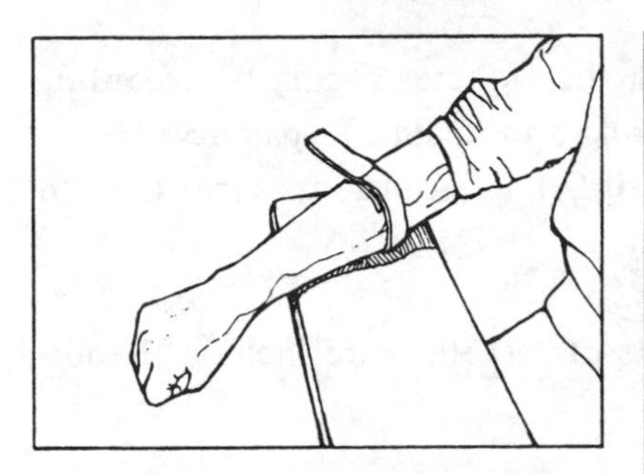

A. Apply tourniquet to mid-forearm, palpate radial pulse, and loosen tourniquet if pulse cannot be felt. Have patient open and close fist for venous distention.

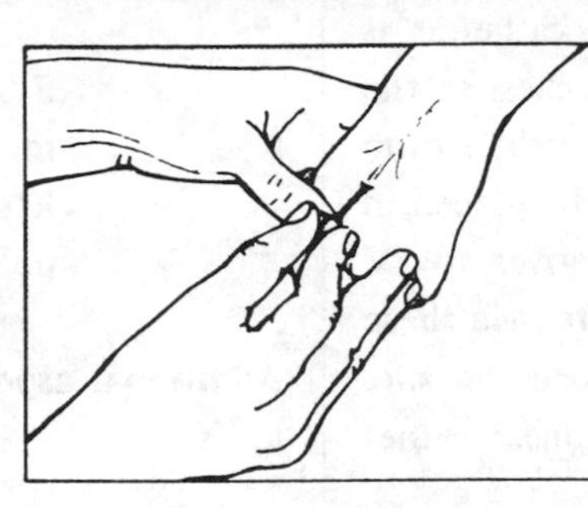

B. Cleanse injection area and hold patient's hand, using thumb to keep skin taut and anchor vein. Place needle in line with vein, bevel up, about one-half in. below proposed entry site.

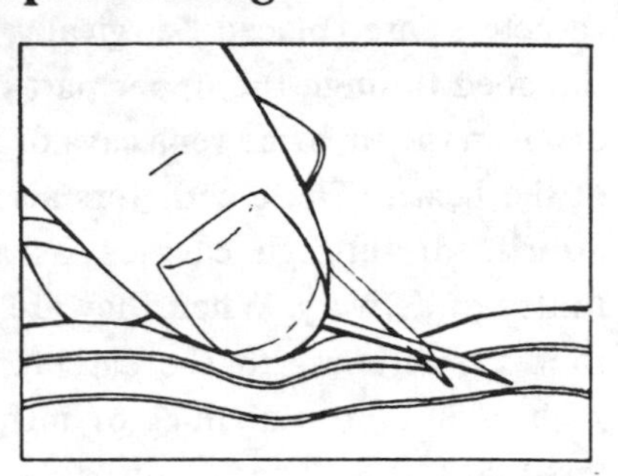

C. Insert needle through skin and tissue at 45° angle, relocate vein, decrease needle angle slightly, and slowly enter vein with a downward then upward motion.

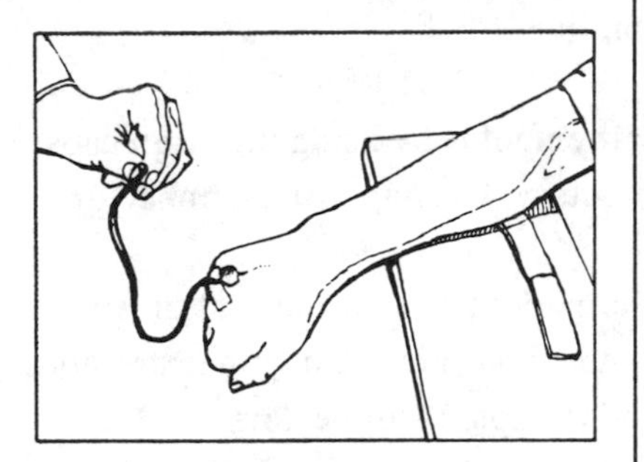

D. Remove tourniquet and tape scalp vein tubing.

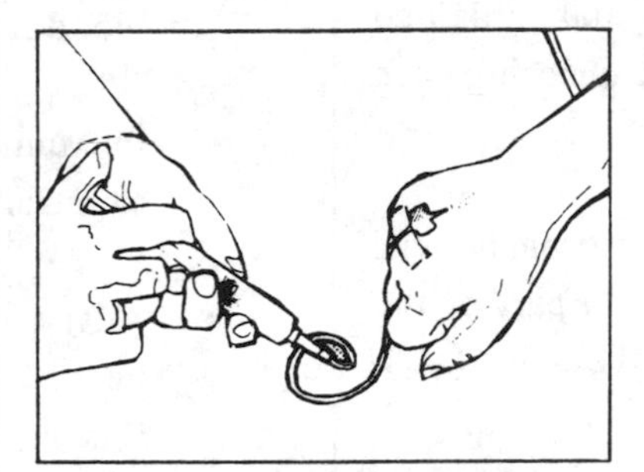

*E. Attach syringe of saline, aspirate to remove air and irrigate.

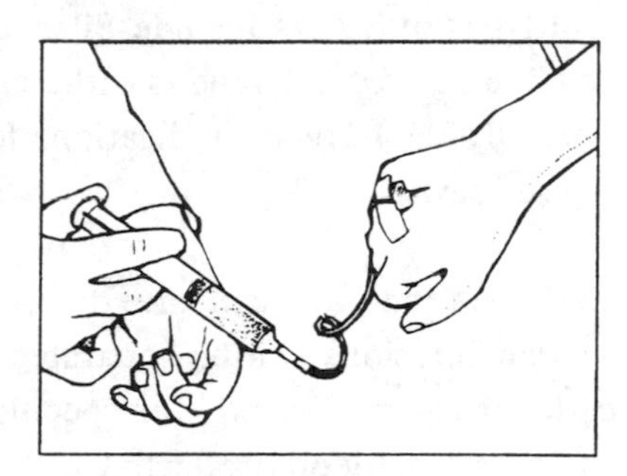

*F. Remove saline syringe, attach chemotherapy syringe, and inject slowly, checking for blood return and swelling.

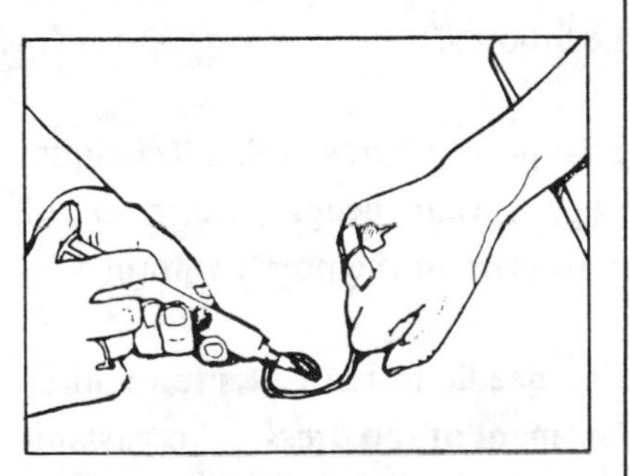

G. Flush catheter with saline solution.

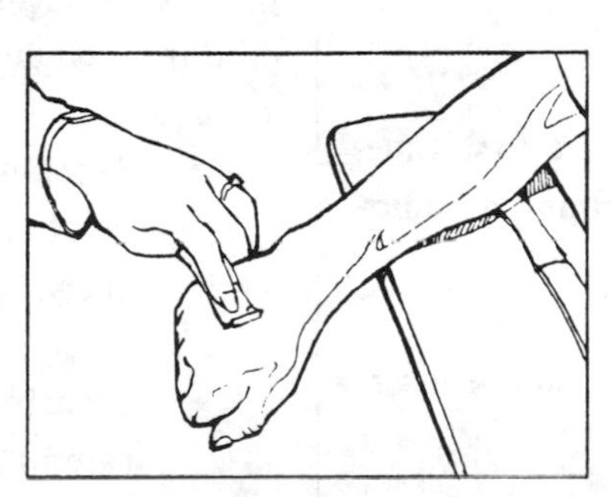

H. Remove needle, apply pressure to prevent bleeding, and apply Band-Aid.

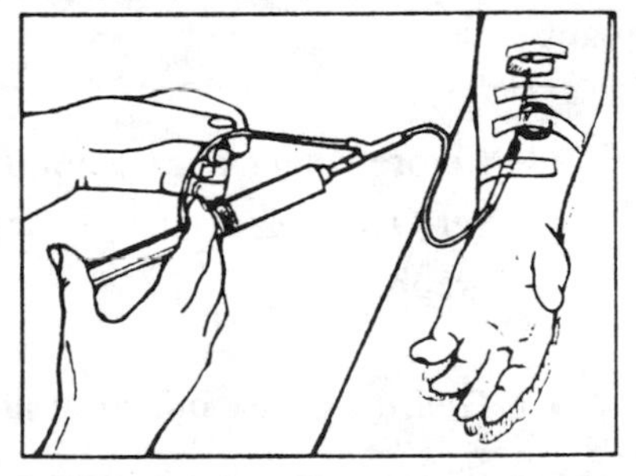

I. If administering agent via side arm of continuously running IV line, establish IV access and freely dripping fluid. Cleanse sidearm, insert needle of syringe with agent, and administer drug, maintaining even pressure.

*E and F demonstrate the two-syringe technique.

Created by Lcdr Judith Ann Killman, BSN, MA, MS, 1990.

obtain blood samples and to administer blood products or total parenteral nutrition.) In general, these catheters are placed surgically; the catheter is threaded through the upper part of the chest so the end is in the superior vena cava or in the right atrium of the heart. (These catheters also can be placed in arteries or through cavities, as alternatives to IV routes of delivery. When they are inserted via these routes, references to the catheter include the site, such as interarterial lines or intraperitoneal catheters.)

Many variations of these catheters are available. Appendix A provides some examples. A few selected proprietary devices are shown there. The following is a general description of types of central catheters. General types of VADs include Silastic atrial catheters, small-gauge central venous catheters, and implanted ports. Table 4-3 gives indications for choosing each type of device.

Catheters and ports can have double or triple lumens so that infusions can be separated or a part of the catheter can be "saved" for specific therapies (such as delivery of blood products.)

Each institution has established policies to care for these catheters and the exit sites. These policies should cover some universal concerns (Tenenbaum, 1989):

- Before using a catheter for the first time, verify its placement by obtaining a radiograph.
- Guard against infection at the site of insertion:
  - Use aseptic technique when manipulating the catheter or changing a dressing of the site of insertion.
  - Check the insertion site for redness, edema, pain, discharge, warmth, and odor, and check the patient for fever or signs of systemic infection.
  - Culture material from the insertion site if you suspect an infection.
  - Flush the catheter regularly, according to policy, to maintain patency. Use a heparin/saline solution, according to policy.

Additional aspects of catheter care include the following:

- Change dressings and care for the insertion site as appropriate.
- Irrigate the VAD (via injection cap, extension set, or T-connector) daily or per protocol after administration of drugs or after blood sampling.
- Prevent air embolus by using injection caps, extension sets with clamps, or T-connectors.
- Advise the patient to use the Valsalva maneuver when you are changing extension sets, injection caps, T-connectors.
- Know how to repair the catheter.

If the VAD is an implantable port, additional considerations include the following:

- Accessing the port requires skilled technique, involving appropriate needle size, angle of entry, and pressure to the port's septum.
- Securing the needle at the exit site requires careful placement of the dressing to cushion the skin and stabilize the entry site.

Intraarterial route. The intraarterial route is a means to deliver high concentrations of chemotherapeutic agents directly to the tumor while decreasing the agents' toxic effects systemically. Catheters can be placed surgically or percutaneously. The catheters usually are connected to an external

Table 4-2

Types of Venous Access Devices and Indications for Their Use

Silastic Atrial Catheters	Small-Gauge Central Venous Catheters	Implanted Ports
Frequent venous access required for blood sampling, blood products, therapy, etc.	Short-term infusion of chemotherapeutic agents (2-3 months)	Single bolus injections of chemotherapeutic agents
Bone marrow transplant recipient	Short-term infusion of vesicant chemotherapeutic agents	Inpatient/outpatient infusion of nonvesicant chemotherapeutic agents
Patient with leukemia	Inpatient/outpatient infusion therapy	Short- or long-term chemotherapy
Single bolus injections of chemotherapeutic agents	Single bolus injections of chemotherapeutic agents	Used for TPN, blood transfusions, fluid replacement, or antibiotics
Total parenteral nutrition (TPN) and antibiotic therapy	Frequent venous access needed for chemotherapy	Infrequent blood sampling required
Short- or long-term infusion of chemotherapeutic agents (vesicant or nonvesicant)	Infrequent blood sampling via peripheral vein	Patient physically unable to care for VAD
Inpatient/outpatient infusion of chemotherapeutic agents	Brief life expectancy	A young child: frequent venous access not required
Significant other or patient capable of caring for device	Significant other or patient capable of caring for device	Cosmesis/patient preference

Source: Goodman, M. (1986). *Cancer: Chemotherapy and care.* Evansville: Bristol-Myers Squibb Oncology Division, Bristol-Myers Squibb Company. Reprinted with permission.

infusion pump or to an implantable access port. This route is used for hepatic artery infusion for metastatic liver disease.

Intracavitary route. The intracavitary route delivers the agent directly to a hollow organ via an indwelling catheter. After the agent has bathed the area, the agent is drained. Bladder or intraperitoneal tumors can be treated in this way.

The intraperitoneal (IP) route is used to treat tumors in the abdominal cavity (e.g., ovarian, colonic).

Table 4-3

Patient Assessment Criteria for a Vascular Access Device

Criteria
Frequency of venous access
Longevity of treatment
Mode of administration
Venous integrity
Patient preference

Low Priority	High Priority
Infrequent venous access	Frequent venous access
Short-term therapy	Long-term indefinite treatment period
	Continous infusion chemotherapy
Intermittent single injections	Home infusion of chemotherapeutic drugs
Administration of nonvesicant/ nonirritating drugs	Administration of vesicant/irritating drugs
No previous IV therapy	Venous thrombosis/sclerosis due to previous IV therapy
Both extremities available	Venous access limited to one extremity
Venous access with two or fewer venipunctures	Prior tissue damage due to extravasation
	Multiple (> 2) venipunctures to secure venous access
Patient does not prefer VAD	Patient prefers VAD

Created by Lcdr Judith Ann Killman, BSN, MA, MS, 1990.

This technique is an adaptation of methods used in peritoneal dialysis. High concentrations of chemotherapeutic agents are delivered to the peritoneal cavity through (a) an implanted port leading to the peritoneal cavity or (b) a catheter (Tenckhoff) inserted through a small incision below the umbilicus. Treatment begins with the delivery of chemotherapeutic agents after the port or catheter has been inserted and the site has healed somewhat. The drugs flow into the peritoneal cavity by gravity from a bottle or bag of dialysis solution. Either the solution is excreted in time by the body, or it is drained from the peritoneal cavity by gravity after a prescribed dwell time. The number of exchanges, the dwell time, and treatment schedules vary.

Complications of IP chemotherapy include abdominal pain because of peritoneal irritation, incomplete drainage of fluid, dialysate solution at a temperature lower than the body temperature, or chemical or bacterial peritonitis.

The intrapleural route is used to introduce certain medications into the pleural cavity via a thoracotomy tube or catheter. The medications cause sclerosis of the pleural lining and thus prevent reaccumulation of fluid in the pleural cavity, generated from the malignancy. Agents used to produce this sclerosis include mechlorethamine, fluorouracil, bleomycin, and doxycycline.

After the sclerosing agent is instilled, the patient usually must change body position every 10 to 15 minutes to allow circulation of the sclerosing agent through the pleural cavity.

Intrathecal route. Because most agents cannot pass the blood-brain barrier, drugs used to treat tumors of the cerebrospinal fluid (CSF) of meninges are delivered through the spinal fluid via a lumbar puncture. (i.e. intrathecal route). Agents that may be used are methotrexate, cytarabine, and thiotepa. In addition to side effects from the agents, adverse effects of this route of treatment are headaches, stiff neck, lethargy, nausea and vomiting, and confusion and seizures.

Ventricular reservoir. A ventricular reservoir is an alternative method used to deliver chemotherapeutic drugs to the CSF. It provides more consistent levels of drug in the cerebrospinal fluid and allows the drug to reach the ventricles of the brain. A device (Figure 4-5, Ommaya reservoir) is surgically implanted SC in the frontal region of the skull over the coronal suture. A hole is burred into the lateral ventricle in the area of the foramen of Monro. The chemotherapeutic agent then is injected through the reservoir. Complications include infection, malfunction of the reservoir because of blockage, and displacement of the catheter. Drugs administered by this route circulate better if the reservoir is pumped. Push down gently with a finger on top of the reservoir several times.

Informed Consent

Many policies on informed consent state that the physician is responsible for obtaining consent from the patient. The nurse shares the responsibility in clarifying and reinforcing information that has been given to the patient. General principles of informed consent include the following (Oncology Nursing Society, 1988):

- The patient has heard a description of and shows an understanding of the therapy he or she is to receive.
- Risks, specifically side effects or toxic reactions, are explained, as well as the benefits of therapy.
- Alternatives to the therapy are explained, including their risks and benefits.
- Consent, either verbal or written, is obtained from the patient and varies with the institution. That consent should become part of the medical record.

In obtaining informed consent, the nurse is the reinforcer, interpreter, and communicator on behalf of the patient. In administering chemotherapy, the nurse's role with regard to informed consent is invaluable.

Safe Handling of Chemotherapeutic Agents

Recommendations and guidelines for handling cytotoxic agents are provided by the Occupational Safety and Health Administration (OSHA) and the National Study Commission on Cytotoxic Exposure. These recommendations do provide a sensible framework for working with such agents. Highlights of the recommendations follow (OSHA, 1986). Any nurse who deals with chemotherapeutic agents should keep abreast of the latest guidelines. Your institution should be able to provide you with the latest recommendations. (Note: These highlights include recommendations only for handling agents. Other recommendations exist for those who prepare, transport, and store the agents.)

- Only registered nurses who have been instructed and designated as qualified in the handling and administration of chemotherapeutic agents should be responsible for administering these agents. Administration should include adher-

Figure 4-5
Ommaya Reservoir

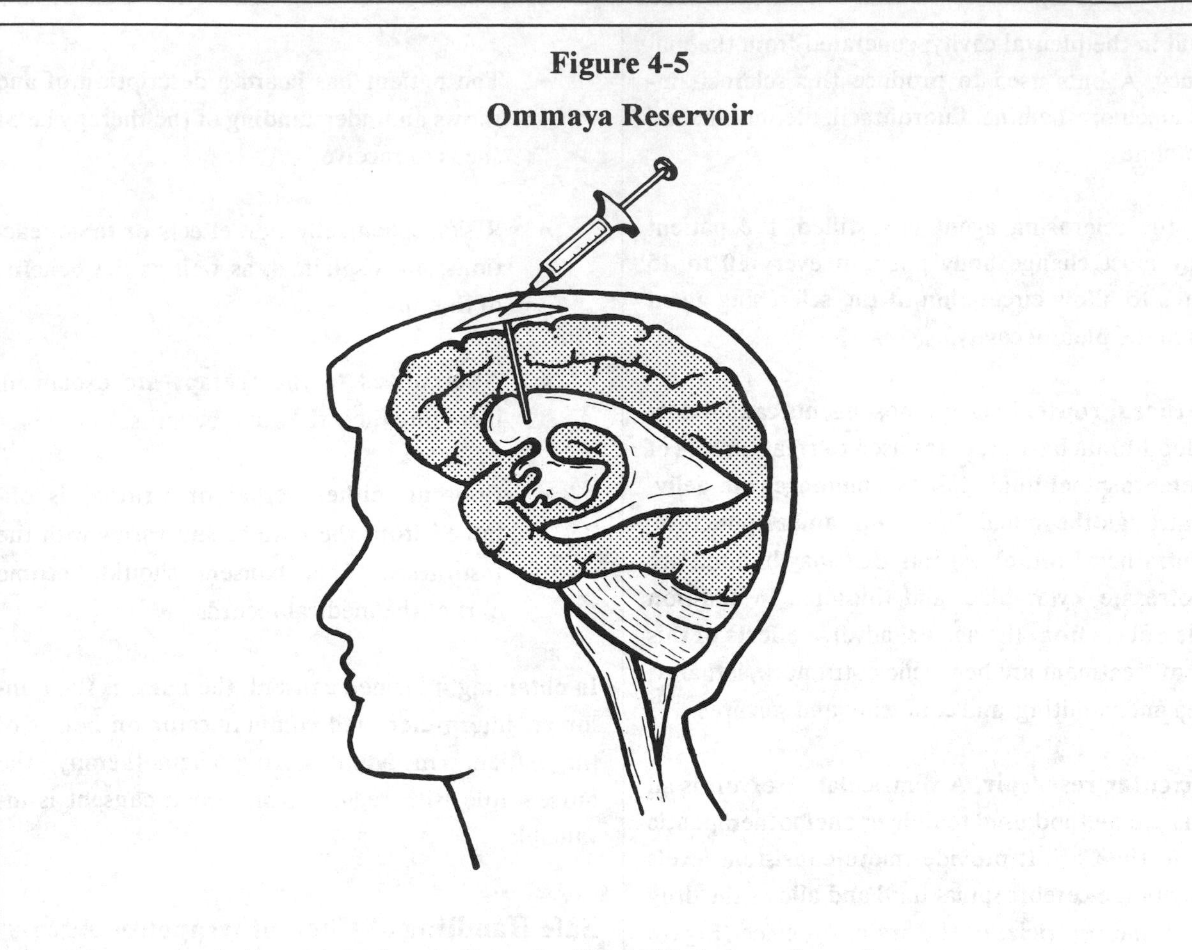

Illustration reproduced with permission from the University of Texas M.D. Anderson Cancer Center.

ence to aseptic technique, safety, and proper disposal of materials and the patient's excreta.

- To ensure safe handling, prepare all cytotoxic agents according to the package insert. If possible, use a class II biological safety cabinet with outside venting of the hood.
- Wear chemo latex gloves and a disposable gown made of lint-free, low-permeability fabric with closed long sleeves and elastic or knit closed cuffs. Tuck the cuffs in under the gloves. (Note: Surgical latex gloves are less permeable to many chemotherapeutic drugs than polyvinyl chloride gloves are. Never use powdered gloves.)
- Wash your hands before putting on gloves and gowns. If your gloves become contaminated, change them immediately.
- Use infusion sets and pumps that have Luer-Lok fittings and tubing and check for signs of leakage during use. (Note: Non-Luer-Lok connections can separate from the pressure of the syringe plunger.)
- Prime the infusion line with the IV solution before adding the chemotherapeutic agent to the solution. If, for some reason, priming is done at the bedside, be even more careful. Priming should be done into a sterile dry gauze in a labeled plastic bag.

When connecting the IV tubing to the IV catheter or maintenance IV line, avoid spilling or aerosolizing the chemotherapeutic agents. Protect both the patient and yourself:

- Use disposable plastic-backed liners under the patient's arm or hand to prevent spillage on the bed.

- Use sterile gauze at the injection site to prevent spillage on the patient.

- Wear recommended protective clothing during administration of chemotherapeutic agents at the bedside.

- Prevent aerosolization of drugs by shielding the needle with sterile gauze when pulling the needle from its cover or IV tubing port.

- Secure the tubing connection site with tape or other device (e.g., Clik-lock).

- Dispose of all materials (e.g. IV bags, tubing, gloves) which have been in contact with the hazardous (cytotoxic) dugs in specially marked hazardous waste (leakproof, puncture proof) containers.

- Have a spill kit accessible.

After the drug has been administered, follow Federal OSHA guidelines for destroying sharps. These guidelines, published in December 1991, recommend that contaminated needles and other sharps not be recapped. Because of the possibility of injury during the process of recapping or otherwise destroying needles and sharps, contaminated products are to be placed intact into disposable containers that meet OSHA guidelines for disposal (OSHA, 1991).

Documentation

Documentation of administration of a chemotherapeutic agent should include the following (OSHA, 1988):

- Location of the IV site (if IV route was used)
- Drugs and dosages administered
- Sequence of drug administration
- Needle type and size (if applicable)
- Amount and type of flushing solution (if applicable)
- Description of site after treatment (if applicable)
- Adverse reactions, if any
- Side effects discussed and experienced
- Reactions to treatment

EDUCATION OF THE PATIENT

Administration of chemotherapy often focuses on the technique of giving agents. This information is important, but it should not outweigh the critical component of teaching the patient. No matter how good the hands-on skill of the nurse, chemotherapy is administered in partnership with the patient. Without a knowledgeable patient, informed consent does not exist, and feedback from the patient about the therapy will not be available. A nurse cannot assume that administration has been safe and effective if the patient cannot provide crucial input about what it feels like when he or she receives the agent. The only expert on side effects is the patient. Explanation of severity, duration, or intensity can come only from the patient.
Therefore, teaching the patient must precede administering the drugs.

A patient's anxiety about and fear of chemotherapy may be related to lack of understanding of the treatment and its side effects. Presenting accurate information about why the therapy is being given and how the patient will know if it is helping will make it easier for the patient to cope with this therapy (Longman, 1990).

The patient's level of understanding and readiness to learn will vary. Many patients cope better if they have a lot of information; others find that too much information is overwhelming. At first, minimize anxiety by describing briefly what can be expected with each treatment, emphasizing the overall benefits of therapy.

Many resources provide information for cancer patients and about treatment options. You may wish to develop standard sources for patients or tailor information that better fits your patients' needs. Sources of patient education materials include the following:

- The American Cancer Society
- Hospital cancer centers
- National Cancer Institute
- Oncology Nursing Society
- Association of Pediatric Oncology Nurses
- Association of Community Cancer Centers
- American Association of Cancer Education
- American Society of Clinical Oncologists
- International Union Against Cancer
- Manufacturers of drugs and devices
- Numerous textbooks and periodicals

For more suggestions, see the suggested reading list or bibliography at the end of the curriculum.

EXAM QUESTIONS

Chapter 4

Questions 16–28

16. Vascular access devices are used to do which of the following?

    a. Administer oxygen
    b. Administer chemotherapy and blood products
    c. Provide total parenteral nutrition
    d. Separate platelets and WBCs

17. Intraperitoneal chemotherapy is used to treat which of the following types of cancer?

    a. Breast cancer
    b. Ovarian cancer
    c. Lung cancer
    d. Leukemia

18. Adverse effects of intrathecal chemotherapy include

    a. Hearing loss
    b. Headaches
    c. Decreased number of neutrophils
    d. Chest pain

19. The nurse's role in administering chemotherapeutic agents includes:

    a. Teaching the patient what to expect during and after administration
    b. Giving the agents in a rushed, hurried environment
    c. Administering chemotherapy before establishing informed consent
    d. Administering chemotherapy before checking the laboratory data

20. What steps can nurses take to limit their exposure to the harmful effects of chemotherapeutic agents during administration?

    a. Wear powdered gloves.
    b. Dispose of materials in unlabeled trash cans.
    c. Wear gloves and gowns.
    d. Allow aerosolization of the agents.

21. Why are chemotherapy latex gloves better than polyvinyl chloride gloves for administration of chemotherapeutic agents?

    a. They can be used with powder.
    b. They are purple.
    c. They are sterile.
    d. They are less permeable to many chemotherapeutic agents.

22. Veins suitable for venipuncture should feel

    a. Smooth and pliable
    b. Hard and sclerotic
    c. Knotty and soft
    d. Edematous and tender

23. Before administering any cytotoxic agent to any patient, the nurse must do which of the following?

    a. Determine if drug can cross the blood-brain barrier.
    b. Review the patient's history of any experiences with chemotherapy.
    c. Change the IV tubing.
    d. Assess the patient's hearing.

24. Steps to protect the patient from spillage or aerosolization of a chemotherapeutic agent during IV administration include

    a. Shielding the needle with sterile gauze when pulling it from its cover or from the IV tubing port
    b. Taping the tubing connection site loosely
    c. Covering the patient's arm or hand with a plastic-backed liner
    d. Using non–Luer-Lok connections

25. Preferred venipuncture sites are

    a. Wrist veins
    b. Cephalic veins
    c. Digital veins
    d. Antecubital fossa

26. What should the nurse do if a nonvesicant agent infiltrates during its administration?

    a. Give epinephrine.
    b. Discontinue the infusion and restart the injection at a different site.
    c. Leave the needle in place and aspirate as much of the residual medication as possible.
    d. Complete the injection.

27. Dosages in chemotherapy are based on

    a. Body surface area
    b. Patient's birthday
    c. Family history
    d. Blood type

28. Complications of intraperitoneal chemotherapy include

    a. Headaches
    b. Stiff neck
    c. Hemorrhage
    d. Peritonitis

CHAPTER 5

SELECTED CHEMOTHERAPEUTIC AGENTS

CHAPTER OBJECTIVE

After completing this chapter, you will be able to name specific chemotherapeutic agents, how they are given, and their side effects.

LEARNING OBJECTIVES

After reading this chapter, you will be able to

1. Identify three chemotherapeutic agents and their range of doses.
2. Highlight precautions to take before administering three different agents.
3. Specify the major side effects of three different chemotherapeutic agents.

This chapter is a brief listing of some of the common chemotherapeutic agents. As a nurse giving these agents, you also should refer to drug information from your institution's pharmacy, other drug reference books, and data supplied by the manufacturer. The listing provides the main characteristics about the agents. To better understand the rationale in giving these drugs, look to other chapters in this curriculum.

Agents are listed in alphabetical order. Generic names appear first, then proprietary or trade names and acronyms. Material in this chapter is based on data from *Cancer Chemotherapy: A Reference Guide* (Tenenbaum, 1989) and *Cancer Chemotherapy: Treatment and Care* (Knobf, Fischer, Welch-McCaffrey, 1984). Dosages and routes are for standard therapies or for those therapies in which the agent is given alone. When giving the agents, check with recent drug sources for specific dosage ranges and protocols.

BLEOMYCIN (BLENOXANE®)

Class: Antitumor antibiotic.

Indications: Squamous cell cancers, lymphomas, testicular cancer.

Special Precautions: Some recommend a test dose of 1–5 units to determine hypersensitivity is recommended. (Sources vary on which route of administration to choose.) Monitor vital signs every 15 minutes for 1 hour before proceeding with prescribed drug order.

Dosage: 10–20 units/m^2, one or two times each week (1 mg = about 1 unit), or 0.25–0.5 units/kg. Cumulative lifetime dose should not exceed 200 units/m^2.

Administration: IV, IM, SC, and by regional arterial infusion. IM or SC injection can cause pain or burning at the injection site.

Side Effects

- Pulmonary changes: Can be manifested as pneumonitis but can progress to pulmonary fibrosis. This toxic reaction is more common in patients who are more than 70 years old. Radiation therapy enhances pulmonary toxic effects. Use pulmonary function tests to monitor changes. Risk is also increased with total cumulative doses > 200mg/m^2.

- Fever and chills: Usually occur 4–10 hours after drug is administered and can last for up to 2 days. Acetaminophen and antihistamines (e.g., diphenhydramine) can control reaction. Consult manufacturer's recommendations for appropriate treatment.

- Stomatitis: Depends on route, dose, duration of infusion.

- Skin hyperpigmentation, cutaneous changes: May occur on palms and fingers. Nail-bed changes (discolored and texture changes) also may occur. Protect the skin from friction, pressure, or extremes of temperature.

BUSULFAN (MYLERAN®)

Class: Alkylating agent.

Indications: Chronic myelogenous leukemia, polycythemia vera, and myeloid metaplasia.

Special Precautions: If the WBC count is high, provide additional hydration to avoid hyperuricemia.

Dosage: 2–10 mg/day (or 1.8 mg/m^2) for 2–3 weeks; maintenance dose is 1–3 mg/day. Stop drug when WBC reaches 10,000–20,000 cells/cu mm.

Administration: Oral.

Side Effects

- Bone marrow suppression: Maximum occurs 14 days after administration begins, and suppression may continue until day 30. Usually dose related.

- Pulmonary changes: Interstitial pulmonary fibrosis may develop after long-term therapy.

- Additional side effects: Nausea and vomiting, diarrhea, glossitis, sterility, generalized skin hyperpigmentation, and testicular or ovarian fibrosis or atrophy. Usually dose related and stops when treatment stops.

CARMUSTINE (BiCNU®) [BCNU]

Class: Nitrosourea.

Indications: Hodgkin's and non-Hodgkin's lymphoma, brain and lung cancers, multiple myeloma.

Special Precautions: Drug can stay in cerebral spinal fluid for as long as 9 hours after administration. During administration, drug can burn at injection site along the vein. Apply ice and/or slow rate to prevent or lessen pain. Some experts advise administering carmustine last if giving multiple agents, to limit irritation to veins.

Dosage: 75–100 mg/m^2 daily for 2 days or 200 mg/m^2 as one dose every 6 weeks.

Administration: Usually given IV over 1–2 hours.

Side Effects

- Nausea and vomiting: Can occur 2–4 hours after administration and can last for 4–6 hours.
- Bone marrow suppression: Maximum occurs 3–5 weeks after administration. Cumulative toxic effects can occur. Thrombocytopenia is usually more severe than leukopenia.
- Pulmonary changes: Toxic effects as fibrosis (with dyspnea, tachypnea, nonproductive cough) can occur 6 months after therapy. Toxic effects also can occur when therapy includes bleomycin or radiation therapy to the chest.
- Hepatic effects: Liver function tests can be abnormal.

CISPLATIN (PLATINOL®) [DDP]

Class: Heavy metal; acts like an alkylating agent.

Indications: Testicular, ovarian, head, and neck cancers; sarcomas; bladder, lung, esophageal, cervical; melanoma.

Special Precautions: Can be neurotoxic, nephrotoxic, and ototoxic. Monitoring and adequate hydration are key to safe delivery. Pre-hydration using at least 1 liter of saline-containing fluid to ensure a urine output of 150 ml/hr. Baseline serum potassium and magnesium and creatinine and creatinine clearance. Giving cisplatin with other nephrotoxic drugs (aminoglycosides, amphotericin B) is not recommended. Thrombophlebitis can occur if drug infiltrates. Do not use aluminum-containing needles or tubing because cisplatin will form a black precipitate with aluminum.

Dosage: 75–120 mg/m^2 every 3–4 weeks or 15–20 mg/m^2 daily for 5 days every 3–4 weeks.

Administration: IV according to various schedules (infusions over 15–20 minutes, 8 hours, or 24 hours). Hydration before and after administration (with or without mannitol or furosemide for diuresis) is recommended to maintain suggested urine output of 100–150 ml/hr.

Side Effects

- Renal toxic effects: Can be cumulative and irreversible, although it is usually reversible.
- Ototological toxic effects: Tinnitis and high-frequency hearing loss.
- Nausea and vomiting: Severe, occuring 1 hour after administration and lasting 24 hours or longer. Antiemetics must be given prior to cisplatin to manage this side effect.
- Bone marrow suppression: Maximum occurs at 1–2 weeks after administration.
- Additional side effects: Replacement of electrolytes, such as magnesium, calcium, potassium, and phosphorus, may be needed.

CYCLOPHOSPHAMIDE (CYTOXAN®) [CTX]

Class: Alkylating agent.

Indications: Hodgkin's and non-Hodgkin's lymphoma; Burkitt lymphoma; multiple myeloma; neuroblastoma; retinoblastoma; rhabdomyosarcoma; Ewing sarcoma; mycosis fungoides; leukemias; and testicular, endometrial, breast, and lung cancers.

Special Precautions: The plasma half-life of cyclophosphamide is 2–9 hours, so the drug can still be present long after administration. If possible, time the administration so that the patient will not have the drug in the bladder overnight.

Dosage: 500–1,500 mg/m^2 IV in divided doses every 3–4 weeks or 60–100 mg/m^2 orally each day.

Administration: IV and oral. Hydration before and after IV administration is important.

Side Effects

- Nausea and vomiting: Occur about 6 hours after administration and can last 8–10 hours or longer. Antiemetics should be given prior to IV administration. Small, light meals; and relaxation methods may also reduce nausea and vomiting.
- Bone marrow suppression: Maximum occurs 7–14 days after administration, with recovery in another 7–10 days.
- Hemorrhagic cystitis: Chemical irritation to the bladder results in hematuria. Efforts to avoid cystitis include hydration (3–4 liters/day), frequent voiding, and eliminating evening administration. If cyclophosphamide is given with doxorubicin, alert the patient that urine may be pink from doxorubicin rather than from blood.
- Alopecia: Can occur 3–4 weeks after treatment begins. Hair will return after treatments stop.
- Nasal stuffiness: With large IV doses, symptoms can include runny eyes, rhinorrhea, and sneezing.
- Sterility: Amenorrhea and depression of sperm count can occur.
- Secondary malignancies: Bladder cancer and acute leukemias have been linked to administration of cyclophosphamide.

CYTARABINE (CYTOSAR-U®) [CYTOSINE, ARABINOSID, ARA-C]

Class: Antimetabolite.

Indications: Acute myelocytic or lymphocytic leukemia, lymphomas.

Special Precautions: Various dosages and schedules are used according to diagnosis.

Dosage: Leukemias: 100 mg/m2 IV each day for 5–10 days or 100 mg/m2 IV or SC every 12 hours for 1–3 weeks. Higher doses (2–3 gms/m^2 every 12 hrs for 6–10 doses) to treat leukemia are common.

Administration: IV. Rapid IV infusion can cause dizziness and somnolence; nausea can be less severe if infusion is slower. Often given via continuous infusion.

Side Effects

- Bone marrow suppression: Maximum usually occurs at 7–14 days after administration. Is related to dose, frequency, and duration of therapy.
- Nausea and vomiting: Increase with higher doses and can last for several hours. Antiemetics offer limited help.
- Hepatic effects: Liver dysfunction occurs but can be reversible.
- Additional side effects: Headache, thrombophlebitis, pulmonary edema, diarrhea, myalgias, rash, malaise, and fever have been reported with higher doses. Conjunctivitis and cerebellar ataxia may occur. When conjunctivitis is anticipated, steroid eyedrops can be given to prevent the occurrence.

DACARBAZINE (DTIC–DOME®) [IMIDAZOLE, CARBOXIMIDE]

Class: Alkylating agent.

Indications: Malignant melanoma, Hodgkin's disease, sarcomas.

Special Precautions: Prevent extravasation. Patients report burning at injection site that will not stop even if infusion rate is decreased. Applying ice to the site may give some comfort.

Dosage: 150–250 mg/m^2 day for 5 days every 4 weeks.

Administration: Slow IV push (2–3 minutes) over 20 minutes as drip, or also, as 2-hour drip. Because of pain and burning at the site, an IV drip is recommended.

Side Effects

- Nausea and vomiting: Higher doses cause more severe signs and symptoms. Over 5-day course, nausea and vomiting can abate over time.
- Flulike syndrome: Patients may experience malaise, headache, and sinus congestion.
- Bone marrow suppression: Appears about 2 weeks after administration.
- Additional side effects: Include metallic taste, photosensitivity, alopecia, rashes, and flushing.

DACTINOMYCIN (COSMEGEN®) [ACTINOMYCIN D]

Class: Antitumor antibiotic.

Indications: Testicular cancer, melanoma, choriocarcinoma, Wilms tumor, neuroblastoma, retinoblastoma, rhabdomyosarcoma, Ewing sarcoma, and Kaposi sarcoma.

Special Precautions: Avoid extravasation. Dactinomycin potentiates the effects of radiation therapy, so dose should be reduced if radiation treatment is given concurrently or at generally the same time.

Dosage: 15–30 mcg/kg for 1 week or 10–15 mcg/kg each day for 5 days.

Administration: Through running IV line.

Side Effects

- Bone marrow suppression: Maximum occurs 10–14 days after administration. Dose limits are imposed because of suppression.

- Nausea and vomiting: Can begin 2–5 hours after administration and can last for 24 hours. With longer courses of therapy, constant severity of nausea and vomiting may be reduced.

- Alopecia: Can begin 7–10 days after administration.

- Dermatological effects: Acnelike papules may develop on the face and may spread to the trunk. Areas previously exposed to radiation may appear red.

- Secondary malignancies: Risk increases in areas previously exposed to radiation.

- Additional side effects: Malaise, stomatitis, diarrhea, anorexia, fatigue, and lethargy.

DAUNORUBICIN (CERUBIDINE®) [DAUNOMYCIN, RUBIDOMYCIN]

Class: Antitumor antibiotic.

Indications: Acute lymphoblastic and myeloblastic leukemia.

Special Precautions: Avoid extravasation. Urine may appear pink for 2 days after administration, so advise patient accordingly.

Dosage: 30–60 mg/ m^2 IV each day for 3 days.

Administration: Through running IV line, over 2–5 minutes. Use extravasation precautions.

Side Effects

- Nausea and vomiting: Can occur during first 24 hours after administration. Patients should receive prophylactic antiemetics.

- Bone marrow suppression: Maximum occurs at 10–14 days after administration; recovery occurs at 3 weeks.

- Alopecia: Complete hair loss occurs about 3–4 weeks after therapy begins.

- Stomatitis: May occur 3–7 days after administration and may worsen.

- Cardiac effects: Irreversible congestive heart failure (CHF) may occur. Lifetime cumulative dose should not exceed 550 mg/m^2 (440 mg/m^2 if previous radiation therapy to chest or treatments with cyclophosphamide). CHF may occur 6 months after treatment has ended.

- Hepatic effects: Abnormalities in liver function (elevated Bilirubin) warrant reduction in dosage.

DOXORUBICIN HYDROCHLORIDE (ADRIAMYCIN®)

Class: Antitumor antibiotic.

Indications: Breast, bladder, thyroid, ovarian, and small-cell lung cancers; acute leukemias; sarcomas; neuroblastomas; Hodgkin's and non-Hodgkin's lymphomas; and Ewing sarcoma.

Special Precautions: Doxorubicin is a vesicant, so avoid extravasation. Flare along the vein during or after administration can occur. Flare can appear as reddening or wheals along the vein. Flare appearance does not mean drug should be discontinued. Doxorubicin is incompatible with dexamethasong, fluorouracil, and heparin.

Dosage: 60–75 mg/m^2 every 3 weeks, through IV push or continuous IV infusion. Because of cardiac toxic effects, cumulative lifetime dose should not exceed 550 mg/m^2 (400 mg/m^2 if radiation therapy or treatment with cyclophosphamide is part of current or previous therapies).

Administration: IV through side port (over 3–5 minutes) in larger veins. Avoid administration via dorsal hand veins or veins near joints.

Side Effects

- Bone marrow suppression: Maximum occurs 10–14 days after administration.

- Nausea and vomiting: Can begin 1–3 hours after administration. Increase with increased dose and with therapies requiring cyclophosphamide. Patient should receive prophylactic antiemetics.

- Stomatitis: Increases with increased doses.

- Cardiac effects: Irreversible CHF may occur. Can usually monitor by determining electrocardiographic (ECG) changes. Left ventricular cardiac ejection fraction is guide to limiting drug.

- Alopecia: Complete hair loss occurs 2–5 weeks after therapy beings. Regrowth of hair can occur a few months after last treatment.

ETOPOSIDE (VePesid®) [VP-16]

Class: Plant alkaloid.

Indications: Lymphomas; acute nonlymphocytic leukemia; small-cell lung cancer; testicular.

Special Precautions: Bronchospasms and hypotension can occur if agent is given too rapidly.

Dosage: 50–100 mg/m^2 each day for 5 days or 125 mg/m^2 every other day for 3 days, then repeat in 4 weeks. Infusion rate must be at least 60 minutes.

Administration: Oral administration is double IV dose. If dose exceeds 200 mg, divide dose by two hours for optimal absorption. Administer over 30–60 minutes through an IV line. Slow rate of infusion can lessen or prevent wheezing or hypotension.

Side Effects

- Bone marrow suppression: Maximum occurs 7–14 days after administration. Can be limited by dose. Recovery occurs by day 20.

- Nausea and vomiting: Are infrequent.

- Alopecia: Will stop once drug is stopped.

- Additional side effects: Fever, chills, and anorexia.

FLUOROURACIL (ADRUCIL®) [5-FLUOROURACIL] [5FU]

Class: Antimetabolite.

Indications: Stomach, colonic, pancreatic, liver, ovarian, breast, bladder.

Special Precautions: Infiltration causes pain and skin changes.

Dosage: 12-15 mg/kg weekly or 12 mg/kg each day for 5 days every 4 weeks or 200-250 mg/m^2 every other day for 4 days; 500-600 mg/m^2 weekly as continuous infusion. Dose reductions are warranted when liver, renal, or bone marrow status is compromised.

Administration: IV push or slow drip (30 minutes to 24 hours). Hepatic arterial infusion can be given for 8-hour period for 5–21 consecutive days.

Side Effects

- Diarrhea: Presence suggests toxic effects; may need to stop therapy or decrease dosage.
- Stomatitis: Presence suggests toxic effects. Can be managed by frequent assessment and diligent mouth care. May need to stop therapy.
- Bone marrow suppression: Maximum occurs 7–14 days after administration.
- Nausea and vomiting: Ususally mild.
- Photosensitivity or dermatological effects: Rash or increased skin pigmentation may occur, especially on areas exposed to sunlight. Use of sunscreens or avoidance of sun can alleviate effects.

FLOXURIDINE (FUDR®)

Class: Antimetabolite.

Indications: Stomach, colonic, liver.

Special Precautions: Intraarterial route is less toxic to system than IV route. Chemical hepatitis is uncommon but can be severe if it occurs; check for abnormalities in levels of alkaline phosphatase and bilirubin. Temporary reduction or discontinuance of the therapy may be warranted.

Dosage: 100–600 mcg/kg each day for 1–6 weeks.

Administration: Intraarterial.

Side Effects

- Nausea and vomiting: Usually mild.
- Additional side effects: Abdominal cramps, pain, diarrhea, and stomatitis may occur.

HYDROXYUREA (HYDREA®)

Class: Miscellaneous. Interferes with DNA; action similar to that of antimetabolites.

Indications: Chronic myelogenous leukemia, acute leukemia, head and neck cancer, melanoma, and ovarian and colonic cancer.

Dosage: 500–3,000 mg daily.

Administration: Oral.

Side Effects

- Bone marrow suppression: Can be sudden.
- Nausea and vomiting: Can be mild to moderate.
- Additional side effects: Stomatitis, constipation, and renal impairment.

IFOSFAMIDE (IFEX®) [ISOPHOSPHAMIDE]

Class: Alkylating agent.

Indications: Non-Hodgkin's lymphoma; sarcoma; lung, ovarian, and testicular cancers.

Special Precautions: Hydration is essential to offset toxic effects to urinary tract. Administer Mesna concurrently as protection.

Dosage: Various, including 50 mg/kg each day (2,000 mg/m^2 each day) for 5 days; 2,400 mg/m^2 each day for 3 days; 5,000 mg/m^2 as single dose. Lower doses are given when ifosfamide is part of combination therapy.

Administration: IV infusion over at least 30 minutes.

Side Effects

- Urinary tract effects: Dose-limiting toxic effects occur. Hematuria is common.
- Nausea and vomiting: With higher doses and IV push, severity increases. Can start a few hours after therapy and continue for as long as 3 days.
- Alopecia: Hair loss occurs within 2–4 weeks.
- Hepatic effects: Elevated levels of serum transaminase and alkaline phosphatase will decrease over time.
- Neurological effects: High doses can contribute to lethargy and confusion, subsiding after drug is excreted.
- Additional side effects: Side effects similar to those of cyclophosphamide have been reported.

ASPARAGINASE (ELSPAR®) [L-asparaginase]

Class: Miscellaneous. Enzyme; Inhibits protein synthesis.

Indications: Acute lymphoblastic leukemia (induction therapy) and lymphoma.

Special Precautions: Patients can be allergic to one form of L-asparaginase but not another. Two different microbiological sources of asparginase are available. The commercially available Elspar® is derived from *E. coli,* and the investigational form is derived from *Erwinia caratovora.* A third type of asparaginase is known as pegaspargase. It is asparaginase bound to polyethyleneglycol. When allergic reaction occurs, symptoms are rapid urticaria, chills, fever, flushing, and hypotension. To prepare for this situation, do the following:

- Give small test dose first.
- Have antidotes, suggested by manufacturer, easily accessible (i.e., epinephrine, diphenhydramine, hydrocortisone).
- Make sure IV line is patent and running.

Dosage: 1,000 IU/kg IV each day for 2–20 days or 6,000 IU/m^2 IM three times a week for 3 weeks. L-asparaginase generally is used as part of a combination therapy.

Administration: IV through running line or IM.

Side Effects

- Allergic reaction: Urticaria may occur after several doses.
- Fever: Usually 1°C (100.4° F) above normal temperature; antipyretics provide relief.
- Nausea and vomiting: May occur immediately after administration.
- Malaise: Increases as therapy continues.
- Hepatic effects: Liver function tests are abnormal during therapy but return to normal when therapy stops.
- Pancreatitis manifested by an increase in amylase and lipase.

LOMUSTINE (CEENU®) [CCNU]

Class: Nitrosourea.

Indications: Brain tumors, Hodgkin's and non-Hodgkin's lymphomas, melanoma, and lung cancers.

Special Precautions: Give 3–4 hours after meals to limit GI toxic effects. If patient vomits within 30 minutes, repeat dose. Delayed vomiting does not warrant repeat dose.

Dosage: 100–130 mg/m^2 every 6 weeks. Dose limited when bone marrow compromised.

Administration: Oral (on empty stomach). Consider administering agent at night.

Side Effects

- Nausea and vomiting: Occur 4–6 hours after administration.
- Bone marrow suppression: Maximum occurs 4–5 weeks after administration and lasts about 2 weeks. Cumulative doses may cause toxic effects.

MECHLORETHAMINE (MUSTARGEN®) [NITROGEN MUSTARD] [HN_2]

Class: Alkylating agent.

Indications: Hodgkin's and non-Hodgkin's lymphoma, mycosis fungoides, malignant effusions, and bronchogenic cancers.

Special Precautions: Avoid extravasation and contact with skin and eyes.

Dosage: 0.4 mg/kg IV or 12–16 mg/m^2 as single agent. In combination therapies, reduced doses can be scheduled on certain days within month's chemotherapy schedule.

Administration: IV infusion or intracavitary. Give IV infusion through side port of rapidly running IV line over about 3 minutes. Administer immediately after preparation. For special conditions, agent can be given topically or intracavitary.

Side Effects

- Nausea and vomiting: Can start as early as 30 minutes after administration and persist for as long as 2 days.

- Bone marrow suppression: Maximum occurs 10–14 days after administration. Continued suppression of bone marrow function can occur because of previous chemotherapy or radiation treatment.

- Skin rashes: Have been reported.

- Thrombophlebitis: Can be painful. Can be managed with warm soaks and pain medication.

- Additional side effects: Include decreased sperm count, irregular menses, and fever.

MEGESTROL (MEGACE®)

Class: Hormone.

Indications: Endometrial, breast, prostatic, and renal cancers.

Special Precautions: Monitor sodium and calcium levels because of fluid retention.

Dosage: 40 mg four times each day for breast cancer. Up to 80 mg four times each day for endometrial cancer.

Administration: Oral.

Side Effects

- Gynecological effects: Bleeding may occur.

- Nausea and vomiting: May be accompanied by stomach cramps.

- Additional side effects: Fluid retention, causing weight gain; skin rash; headaches; and some jaundice.

METHOTREXATE (MEXATE®) [MTX]

Class: Antimetabolite.

Indications: Acute leukemia; sarcomas; breast, lung, and head and neck cancers; lymphoma; and mycosis fungoides.

Special Precautions: Methotrexate is largely excreted through the kidney unchanged, so patients need to have good kidney function. Moreover, when doses of 1.0–7.5 g/m^2 are used, alkalinization of the urine (with bicarbonate) is necessary before and after administration so that the weak acid of methotrexate is offset. (Without alkalinization, crystals can develop in the kidney.)

Methotrexate binds to serum albumin. Avoid drugs that bind to serum albumin, which would displace methotrexate from the plasma protein. Examples of these albumin-binding drugs are sulfonamides, salicylates, phenytoin, tetracycline, and phenylbutazones. Methotrexate in high doses can be given with folinic acid rescue (leucovorin), as the folinic acid prevents the toxic effects of the methotrexate. Timing of the rescue is crucial; usually it is begun 24 hours after methotrexate is given.

Dosage: Dosage range is large: 30–40 mg/m^2 IV each week or; 100–750 mg/m^2 with leucovorin rescue—(folinic acid). (Frequency of dose depends on protocol.)

Administration: Oral, IV, IM, SC, and intrathecal. Usually given IV. As drug dosage increases, so should period of infusion (IV push for doses less than 150 mg; IV drip for 6 to 36 hours for doses of 150 mg or greater).

Side Effects

- Bone marrow suppression: Maximum occurs 7–14 days after administration.
- Stomatitis: Serves as a warning sign that dosages should be decreased or therapy stopped.
- Nausea and vomiting: Mild to moderate; occur frequently.
- Renal effects: For reasons described in precautions, make sure kidney function is maintained, urine alkalinized for high doses.
- Pulmonary effects: Cough, fever, infiltrates can occur but disappear within 1 week.
- Hepatic effects: Regular liver function studies indicate if fibrosis might be developing.

MITOMYCIN (MUTAMYCIN®)

Class: Antitumor antibiotic.

Indications: GI, breast, lung, cervical, and bladder cancers.

Special Precautions: Avoid extravasation.

Dosage: 2 mg/m^2 each day for 5 days, skip 2 days, then administer for 5 more days. Also, 15 mg/m^2 or 20 mg/m^2 every 6–8 weeks. When used with other agents, doses are lower.

Administration: IV push through rapidly running IV line.

Side Effects

- Nausea and vomiting: Begin 1–2 hours after administration. Vomiting can subside in 3–4 hours. Nausea may continue for 2–3 days. Encourage hydration and other means to manage nausea and vomiting.
- Bone marrow suppression: Maximum occurs 4–5 weeks after administration and may last 2–3 weeks. Lower doses can limit suppression. Suppression can be cumulative.
- Malaise: Occurs universally; related to how long drug is given.
- Pulmonary effects. Interstitial pneumonitis or pulmonary fibrosis can occur.
- Additional side effects: Rise in creatinine levels, alopecia, stomatitis, diarrhea, and fever.

MITOXANTRONE (NOVANTRONE®) [DHAD]

Class: Antitumor antibiotic.

Indications: Acute nonlymphocytic leukemia, acute lymphocytic leukemia, chronic myelocytic leukemia in blast phase, lymphoma, and breast cancer.

Special Precautions: Patient's urine may appear green because mitoxantrone is blue. Also, during infusion, vein may appear blue.

Dosage: 4–12 mg/m^2 each day for 5 days, every 3 weeks.

Administration: IV infusion over 15–30 minutes through running IV line. Flush IV line after administration to avoid burning or stinging at injection site.

Side Effects

- Bone marrow suppression. Maximum occurs 7–14 days after administration. Can be controlled by limiting dose.
- Stomatitis: Mild but common.
- Nausea and vomiting
- Cardiac effects: CHF may develop in patients who have been treated with anthracyclines (Adriamycin®, daunorbicin).

PLICAMYCIN (MITHRACIN®) [MITHRAMYCIN]

Class: Antitumor antibiotic.

Indications: Testicular cancer, Paget disease, hypercalcemia related to malignancy.

Special Precautions: Avoid extravasation.

Dosage: For testicular cancer: 25–50 mcg/kg every other day for three to eight doses, until toxic effects develop.

Administration: Slow IV infusion over 4–6 hours to reduce toxic effects to GI tract.

Side Effects

- Nausea and vomiting: Occur about 6 hours after infusion and last for another 12–24 hours.
- Bone marrow suppression: Bleeding is especially common. Monitor for epistaxis, ecchymosis, petechiae. If symptoms persist, drug should be stopped.
- Additional side effects: Stomatitis, fever, headache, and drowsiness.

PREDNISONE (DELTASONE®, ORASONE®)

Class: Hormone (glucocorticoid).

Indications: Leukemia, lymphomas, mycosis fungoides, multiple myeloma, Hodgkin's disease.

Special Precautions: Can affect blood glucose, sodium, potassium, calcium. Can mask infections. Limit gastric irritation by administering drug with milk or food. Use antacids or H_2 blockers (cimetidine) to limit gastric irritation. Taper dosage if therapy has been stopped.

Dosage: 40–100 mg/m^2 each day

Administration: Oral and IV. If administering IV, use slow infusion to avoid irritation of veins.

Side Effects

- Sodium and fluid retention
- Additional side effects: Over time, include glaucoma, cataracts, osteoporosis, mood swings,

muscle weakness or cramping, increased appetite.

PROCARBAZINE (MATULANE®)

Class: Miscellaneous. (Alkylation; inhibits DNA and RNA synthesis)

Indications: Hodgkin's and non-Hodgkin's lymphoma and bronchogenic cancers.

Special Precautions: Procarbazine can act as a weak monamine oxidase inhibitor. If the patient takes with foods containing tyramine (beer, yogurt, brewer's yeast, wine, cheese, pickled herring, chicken liver), patients can experience sudden hypertension, headaches, or intracranial bleeding. Moreover, agent interacts with sympathomimetic amines (epinephrine, amphetamine) or antidepressants (amitriptyline), causing severe reaction. Procarbazine may cause patients to have symptoms of CNS depression. Avoid administering additional CNS depressants.

Dosage: 50–200 mg daily. Lower doses are prescribed for patients whose liver, kidney, or bone marrow status is compromised.

Administration: Oral.

Side Effects

- Nausea and vomiting: Can be limited by dose. Avoid antihistamine-related antiemetics.
- Bone marrow suppression: Maximum occurs 14-21 days after administration. Can be limited by dose.
- Secondary malignancies: Acute leukemia may develop after treatment with procarbazine.

MERCAPTOPURINE (PURINETHOL®) [6MP]

Class: Antimetabolite.

Indications: Acute leukemia (maintenance therapy) and chronic myelogenous leukemia.

Special Precautions: May need to administer allopurinol with 6MP. Dose of 6MP will be lowered when allopurinol is given also.

Dosage: 100 mg/m^2 each day.

Administration: Oral.

Side Effects

- Bone marrow suppression: Occurs 7 days after administration begins, with recovery at 14 days.
- Hepatic effects
- Additional side effects: Nausea and vomiting, stomatitis, diarrhea, skin eruptions, rash, and hyperuricemia.

TAMOXIFEN (NOLVADEX®)

Class: Hormone.

Indications: Advanced breast cancer in postmenopausal estrogen-receptor–positive women, and more.

Special Precautions: Can cause bone or tumor pain shortly after administration. Analgesias can control discomfort.

Dosage: 10–20 mg twice each day.

Administration: Oral.

Side Effects

- Nausea and vomiting
- Bone marrow suppression
- Gynecological effects: Bleeding and hot flashes. Rarely uterine cancer.
- Occular effects: With high doses, blurred vision, retinopathy may occur.

THIOTEPA [TRIETHYLENE THIOPHOSPHORAMIDE]

Class: Alkylating agent.

Indications: Breast and ovarian cancers and Hodgkin's disease, bladder cancer.

Special Precautions: Pain may occur at the infusion site. If patient is receiving thiotepa through the bladder, encourage changes in body position.

Dosage: 60 mg in instillation of 60 ml once each week; 8 mg/m^2 (0.2 mg/kg) IV each day for 5 days; 30–60 mg IV, IM, or SC once each week.

Administration: IV, IM, SC, and IP for bladder carcinoma.

Side Effects

- Bone marrow suppression: Maximum occurs 7–28 days after administration. Toxic effects are dose limiting.
- Nausea and vomiting: Can worsen with higher doses.
- Additional side effects: Headaches and fever. Allergic reactions include hives and bronchoconstriction.

VINBLASTINE (VELBAN®)

Class: Plant alkaloid.

Indications: Hodgkin's and non-Hodgkin's lymphoma; testicular, head and neck, and breast cancers; renal carcinomas; and Kaposi sarcoma.

Special Precautions: Avoid extravasation. Drug is light-sensitive, so cover infusion bags.

Dosage: 6.0 mg/m^2 IV each week, with lower doses given as first dose.

Administration: IV. Administer over 1 minute through side port of IV line.

Side Effects

- Bone marrow suppression: Maximum occurs 4–10 days after administration.
- Thrombocytopenia: Can be more pronounced if patient has had previous radiation therapy or chemotherapy.
- Neurological effects: Mild peripheral neuropathies and constipation can occur.
- Skin rash: Can occur.

VINCRISTINE (ONCOVIN®) [VCR]

Class: Vinca alkaloid.

Indications: Acute leukemia; Hodgkin's and non-Hodgkin's lymphomas; brain, testicular, breast, and cervical cancers; Wilms tumor; neuroblastoma; and rhabdomyosarcoma.

Special Precautions: Avoid extravasation.

Dosage: 0.4–1.4 mg/m^2 each week. Doses for adults should not exceed 2.0 mg.

Administration: IV. Administer over 1 minute via sidearm of IV line.

Side Effects

- Neurological effects: Vincristine is very toxic to nerve fibers. This can cause hand and feet paresthesias, decreased deep tendon reflexes, ptosis, foot drop, constipation, and paralytic ileus. Regular monitoring and prevention of these complications is warranted (e.g., exercises, laxatives). Reversal of signs and symptoms can occur but may take many months.
- Alopecia: Can occur.
- Additional side effects: Jaw pain, metallic taste in mouth, and hoarseness.

EXAM QUESTIONS

Chapter 5

Questions 29–45

29. One chemotherapeutic agent that can cross the blood-brain barrier is

    a. 5FU
    b. Vinblastine
    c. Testosterone
    d. Carmustine

30. Risk factors for the development of stomatitis include

    a. Chemotherapy protocol that includes 5FU
    b. Hyperthermia
    c. Surgery to the bowel
    d. Use of steroids

31. Special precautions should be taken when administering doxorubicin (Adriamycin) to prevent

    a. Extravasation
    b. Hypotension
    c. Hemorrhagic cystitis
    d. Dehydration

32. One side effect of vincristine is

    a. Neurotoxic effects
    b. Severe nausea and vomiting in 1 to 2 hours
    c. Renal toxic effects
    d. Bronchospasm immediately after infusion

33. Maximal bone marrow suppression (nadir) occurs how many days after administration of methotrexate?

    a. 7–14
    b. 8
    c. 10
    d. 3–6

34. Nonvesicant chemotherapeutic agents include

    a. Carmustine, mitomycin, bleomycin
    b. 5FU, vinblastine, streptozocin
    c. Methotrexate, cisplatin, thiotepa
    d. Asparaginase, dacarbazine, vincristine

35. Doxorubicin causes maximal bone marrow suppression how many days after administration?

    a. 6–8
    b. 16–18
    c. 10–14
    d. 21–28

36. One example of a hormone is

    a. Vincristine
    b. Prednisone
    c. 5FU
    d. 6-Thioguanine

37. What drug is administered with ifosfamide to prevent urinary tract damage?

   a. Mesna
   b. Vitamin B
   c. Tamoxifen
   d. Aspirin

38. Cisplatin is associated with which of the following side effects?

   a. No nausea or vomiting
   b. Nephrotoxic effects
   c. Improved hearing
   d. Increased sense of smell

39. L-asparaginase may do which of the following?

   a. Result in kidney damage
   b. Be given intrathecally
   c. Cause an allergic reaction
   d. Lower the body temperature

40. Megace® is classified as

   a. An alkylating agent
   b. A hormone
   c. An antimetabolite
   d. A nitrosurea

41. Cisplatin is associated with which of the following toxic effects?

   a. Renal toxic effects
   b. Pulmonary fibrosis
   c. Hyperpigmentation
   d. Hypertension

42. Side effects of treatment with 5FU include

   a. Extravasation
   b. Stomatitis
   c. Headaches
   d. Blood in the urine and stool

43. The maximal dose for adults for vincristine is

   a. 0.5 mg/m^2
   b. 2 mg
   c. 8 mg/m^2
   d. 20 mg/m^2

44. Which of the following statements about methotrexate is correct?

   a. It is an alkylating agent.
   b. It is sometimes given with folinic acid (Leucovorin), which serves as a rescue.
   c. It has a very small dosage range.
   d. It is an agent that infrequently causes stomatitis.

45. Prednisone has a tendency to make patients experience

   a. Decreased appetite
   b. Nerve pain
   c. Mood swings
   d. Dehydration

CHAPTER 6

MANAGEMENT OF PATIENTS

CHAPTER OBJECTIVE

After completing this chapter, you will be able to describe side effects of chemotherapy and how they might be managed.

LEARNING OBJECTIVES

After reading this chapter, you will be able to

1. Identify five side effects of chemotherapy.
2. Define bone marrow suppression.
3. Describe how the side effects of stomatitis, constipation, and nausea and vomiting might be managed.
4. Describe three aspects of management of extravasation.
5. Describe three ways to address psychosocial needs of patients receiving chemotherapy.

The nurse who administers chemotherapeutic agents is responsible not only for giving the agent safely but also for helping to manage the care of the patient who has received the agent. Because chemotherapy affects both normal and malignant cells, side effects often can be overwhelming.

Two general categories of adverse effects can occur when chemotherapy is given. The first is side effects resulting from damage to the body's rapidly dividing cells. Examples of cells affected are cells from the bone marrow, hair follicles, cells of the GI tract, and cells that make up reproductive organs or their products. The second is side effects unrelated to the cell cycle but dependent on how the agent is toxic to cells or tissues. These toxic effects can cause organs to malfunction. Examples are the cardiac toxic effects of doxorubicin and the pulmonary toxic effects of bleomycin. Physicians often choose dosages that approach but do not reach toxic levels.

Side effects that seem to receive the most attention are those related to damage to rapidly dividing cells (GI, skin, and bone marrow cells). New cells to replace those cells that have died cannot be reproduced quickly enough. Therefore, this period of aborted cell growth and duplication is especially critical.

This chapter discusses some of the adverse reactions and toxic effects caused by the major chemotherapeutic agents. It also deals with extravasation and anaphylaxis and briefly reviews psychosocial responses as part of the management of patients who are receiving chemotherapy.

BONE MARROW SUPPRESSION

Most chemotherapeutic agents cause some degree of bone marrow suppression (also called myelosuppression): the elimination of functioning bone marrow cells or a decrease in their number. This leads to decreases in the number of WBCs, platelets, and red blood cells (RBCs). The severity of myelosuppression often depends on the dosage and the schedule of administration of the drug. The timing of the suppression can be predicted.

Leukopenia

Leukopenia is a decrease in the total number of circulating WBCs. Because the life span of the leukocyte is brief (12 hours), leukopenia occurs frequently in patients receiving chemotherapy. The normal WBC count is 5,000–10,000 cell/cu mm. When the WBC count drops to the range of 2,500–3,000 cells/cu mm, chemotherapy may be reduced or withheld.

With most myelosuppressive agents, the WBC nadir (or lowest level) occurs 7–14 days after administration of the agent. The next dose of chemotherapy is not administered until bone marrow recovery has occurred. Before the next administration, the WBC count and differential are checked to be sure they are within acceptable limits. The patient should be afebrile and have no signs of infection. A slight infection can lead quickly to sepsis or pneumonia in the immunosuppressed patient.

In counseling patients who are expected to become leukopenic, advise them that their WBC count may decrease after each session of chemotherapy. Inform them that the count usually returns to normal before the next scheduled dose and that if the WBC count is not at an acceptable level, the next dose may be delayed or skipped. Teach the patient how to guard against infection:

- Maintain integrity of mucous membranes and skin.
- Maintain adequate nutrition and fluid intake.
- Avoid persons who have infections.
- Report immediately any signs of infection.
- Maintain personal hygiene.
- Get adequate rest and exercise.

A good indication of the patient's actual ability to fight infection is the differential part of the WBC count known as the absolute granulocyte count (AGC). The AGC is the number of WBCs that are neutrophils (segs bands). (Segs are more mature neutrophils. Bands are less mature neutrophils.) This number provides a more accurate indication of WBCs available to fight infection. The normal AGC is 3,000–7,000 cells/cu mm. Numbers less than 1,000 indicate granulocytopenia. When the AGC is less than 1,500, the patient's status is considered guarded. When the AGC is less than 1,000, the patient is at severe risk for infection.

If an infection develops, the WBC count tends to drop further. Sometimes it may be necessary to administer broad-spectrum antibiotics. Appropriate tests may reveal the source of infection.

Other measures to protect the patient during this risky time include strict handwashing by health care workers before contact with the patient and the daily assessment of any IV sites for possible inflammation.

Patients who are profoundly suppressed should wear a face mask when they leave their hospital room and should not come in contact with persons who have colds or other infections. To reduce the risk of bacterial sources, keep equipment at the bedside rather than carrying it from room to room. At some institutions, plants and flowers may not be kept at the bedside and diet may not include fresh fruits and vegetables because they may harbor bacteria. Take temperatures orally instead of rectally because of the risk of perirectal abscess.

Thrombocytopenia

Thrombocytopenia (a decrease in the number of platelets in the bone marrow) may occur in tandem with leukopenia. Normal platelet counts are 140,000–440,000 cells/cu mm. The risk of spontaneous bleeding occurs when the platelet count falls to less than 20,000 cells/cu mm. A high risk of hemorrhage exists when the platelet count is less than 20,000 cells/cu mm, and hospitalization of the patient may be necessary. When the platelet count is less than 10,000 cells/cu mm, fatal CNS or GI hemorrhaging can occur.

Instruct patients who are receiving a drug known to suppress the platelet count to report the following findings immediately:

- Bleeding gums
- Increased bruising
- Petechiae
- Purpura, especially on lower extremities
- Hypermenorrhea
- Tarry colored stools, blood in urine, or coffee-ground emesis

Teach the patients to protect themselves against bruising or falling. Also give them a list of drugs that tend to disrupt platelet formation and function.

Anemia

Anemia is a reduction in the concentration of hemoglobin and the number of circulating RBCs. With this deficiency, tissues may become hypoxic because the ability of cells to carry oxygen has been impaired. Anemia is indicated by laboratory findings of decreased hemoglobin, hematocrit, or RBC counts.

Initial signs of anemia are fatigue, headache, dizziness, fainting, and dyspnea on exertion (shortness of breath). Irritability is also a common complaint. Loss of color in the nail beds and the palms of the hands also may indicate anemia.

Dehydration may raise the hematocrit, thus masking the anemia. Normal hemoglobin is 13–16 g/dl in males and 12–15 g/dl in females. A hemoglobin of 9.5 g/dl is tolerated by most patients, with some complaints of fatigue and hypothermia. However, patients with a hemoglobin less than 8 g/dl may become uncomfortable and feel short of breath. Severe anemia can lead to hypotension and myocardial infarction.

If the patient has known tumor involvement of the bone marrow, a low hemoglobin is expected. In this case, chemotherapy may actually cause an increase in the hemoglobin because RBC production can increase once the tumor cells in the marrow die.

Patients who have a sudden drop in hemoglobin may be hemorrhaging. The risk of bleeding increases if the patient is also thrombocytopenic. If the hemoglobin concentration drops gradually, and no cause for bleeding can be identified, the patient may have chronic anemia, and care should be supportive. Of course, pacing of activities is important, along with adequate nutrition emphasizing proteins and calories. Of equal importance is addressing the patient's level of comfort, mood, and other feelings (e.g., anxiety and stress).

Nadir

When blood cell counts have reached their lowest point, bone marrow suppression is at its maximum. During this low point, or nadir, the patient is at most risk for infection and hemorrhaging. Therefore, the administration of chemotherapy usually is designed to coincide with the recovery of the bone marrow;

drugs usually are not given during the nadir. A list of approximate nadirs for specific agents is listed in Table 6-1. Despite efforts to schedule chemotherapeutic agents at an optimal time of bone marrow recovery, infection and bleeding associated with myelosuppression are a common cause of death in cancer patients.

In general, agents such as some of the antimetabolites that affect certain phases of the cell cycle are associated with a swiftly occurring nadir and a rapid recovery. Agents, such as the nitrosoureas, that are not phase specific, are associated with delayed bone marrow recovery.

STOMATITIS

Stomatitis (oral mucositis) occurs when rapidly dividing epithelial cells in the mouth, which have been damaged during a course of chemotherapy, slough off or become inflamed. Stomatitis can occur when the tissue is exposed to physical injury through radiation therapy; surgery of the head or neck; or microbial infections, which occur more frequently in immunosuppressed patients. Moreover, stomatitis may increase when patients' nutritional status is compromised, and they may be more susceptible to oral mucosal damage during this time.

The best way to manage stomatitis is to prevent it. Rinsing the mouth frequently with saline or fresh water can minimize it. Once it has occurred, management options depend on its severity. Stomatitis can be graded as follows:

- Grade I: Reddening
- Grade II: Small patches of ulceration
- Grade III: White patches over 15% of oral mucosa
- Grade IV: Ulcerations and bleeding

Stomatitis generally occurs 5–7 days after chemotherapy and persists up to 10 days, depending on the treatment. Reassure patients that the signs are temporary, and instruct them to continue oral hygiene even though it may be painful. If oral hygiene stops or is not thorough, stomatitis can worsen.

Patients with low-grade stomatitis should brush their teeth with a soft-bristled toothbrush and a nonabrasive toothpaste at least every 4 hours and always after eating. Gentle flossing with unwaxed dental floss is recommended. Mouthwash with 1/4-strength hydrogen peroxide and warm water is warranted only if debriding of ulcerations is necessary.

Grades III and IV stomatitis cause difficulty in eating and in maintaining fluid intake. Dehydration can occur, especially if the patient also has diarrhea and nausea and vomiting. If pain is severe, systemic analgesics may be necessary.

Oral hygiene is difficult to maintain because of pain. Oral pain can be relieved by using analgesics or local anesthetics. Rinsing the oral cavity with viscous lidocaine 15 minutes before cleaning it may help. If brushing with a soft brush causes bleeding, have the patient use a sponge or swab.

Lip care should include gentle cleansing. The lips then can be coated with petroleum jelly.

If oral candidiasis (a fungal infection) develops, instruct the patient to swish and swallow an oral suspension of Mycostatin (nystatin) or other antifungal agent at least three times daily after oral hygiene procedures. Ketoconazole (Nizoral) is an oral preparation to prevent or control stomatitis. Clotrimazole (troches) also can be administered.

Stomatitis is often caused or complicated by reactivation of herpes simplex. Therefore, administration of acyclovir may lessen severity and promote healing.

Table 6-1
Myelosuppression*

Drug	WBC Nadir (Days)	WBC Recovery (Days)	Platelet Nadir (Days)	Comment
Asparaginase	NA	NA	NA	Myelosuppression is rarely a problem
Bleomycin	NS	NS	NS	NS
Busulfan	11-30	24-54	NA	
Carmustine	35-42	42-56	28-35	Cumulative delayed, prolonged myelosuppression
Chlorambucil	7-14	NA	7-14	
Cisplatin	7-10	NA	7-10	
Cyclophosphamide	8-14	18-25	10-25	Platelet sparing
Cytarabine	12-14	22-24	22-24	Somewhat platelet sparing
Dacarbazine	10–14	21–28	14-28	
Dactinomycin	15	22-25	10-14	
Daunorubicin	10-14	21	10-14	Profound myelosuppression
Doxorubicin	14	22-25	14	
Etoposide	7-14	21	NS	
5-Fluorouracil	7-14	20-30	7-17	
Hydroxyurea	2-10	21	NA	May spare platelets
Ifosfamide	6-11	20	NA	Platelet sparing
Lomustine	40-50	60	28	Cumulative delayed, prolonged myelosuppression
Mechlorethamine	7-15	14-28	10-14	
Melphalan	10-12	NA	7-14	
6-Mercaptopurine	7	14-21	5-12	
Methotrexate	7-14	14-21	5-12	
Plicamycin	NA	NA	NA	Myelosuppression not usually dose limiting
Mitomycin	21-25	28-42	30	Cumulative prolonged myelosuppression
Mitotane	NA	NA	NA	Myelosuppression rarely dose limiting
Procarbazine	25-36	35-50+	28	Prolonged, delayed myelosuppression
Streptozocin	NA	NA	NA	Myelosuppression not usually dose limiting
6-Thioguanine	8-12	21	8-12	
Thiotepa	14-28	28	14-28	
Vinblastine	5-9	14-21	4-10	Somewhat platelet sparing
Vincristine	3-5	7	NA	Marrow sparing
Vindesine	7	14	7	Platelet sparing

WBC = white blood cell count **NA = not applicable** **NS = not significant**

* Depended on dosage and schedule of administration

Created by Lcdr Judith Ann Killman, BSN, MA, MS, 1990.

NAUSEA AND VOMITING

Chemotherapy often is associated with nausea and vomiting. This situation can be managed so that patients can tolerate therapy. Management of this side effect is important because some patients have chosen to stop chemotherapy rather than continue to experience nausea and vomiting.

Both the physiological and emotional factors related to this side effect should be considered before chemotherapy is administered. If an agent is known to cause significant nausea and vomiting, administer appropriate antiemetics before treatment and on a regular basis during and after treatment. Although each patient's reaction is different, all patients and their families should be told that this side effect can occur but that it can be managed.

Nausea and vomiting can occur when the brain's vomiting center and chemoreceptor trigger zone (CTZ), both located in the medulla, are stimulated. The vomiting center is a motor and a reflex center that can be stimulated by afferent fibers from the GI tract, the vestibular apparatus in the inner ear, and the cerebral cortex. Chemotherapeutic agents can stimulate the CTZ directly, thereby activating the vomiting center. However, the primary mechanism of chemotherapy-induced nausea and vomiting is thought to involve the release of serotonin from cells of the GI tract. The released serotonin interacts with serotonin receptors on the afferent fibers in the GI tract which in turn stimulate the CT2. Drugs which block these receptors (e.g., ondansetron, granisetron) are the most effective antiemetics. Table 6-2 lists the emetogenic potential of some common chemotherapeutic agents.

Other ways to help the patient control nausea and vomiting include continually evaluating the effectiveness of various methods used to reduce their severity. Continual assessment helps the patient find the most effective combination of drugs or other methods. Often patients can identify the regimen that works best for them. For example, some patients prefer a dark, quiet environment where they can be isolated from others and relax before they receive chemotherapy.

Anticipatory nausea and vomiting can be a separate but related reaction to the emetic potential of some chemotherapeutic agents. Patients can have a severe nausea or vomiting response to just the idea of chemotherapy or its related sensations of odor or color. Often the triggers that set off this response have nothing to do with the chemotherapy itself. The sight of a hospital, the memory of the sensation of the nurse administering the chemotherapy, or any associated experience to the treatment can create a conditioned, emetic response for the patient. Lorazepam, a benzodiazepine, can produce amnesia and lessen anticipatory emesis.

Once again, the best way to treat this side effect is to prevent it from happening in the first place. The initial experience of a patient to chemotherapy is crucial in eliminating emetic triggers. Patients who are especially at risk for anticipatory nausea and vomiting are those who are susceptible to it. For example, those who have a history of motion sickness are at increased risk. Patients who are highly anxious are also more likely to experience anticipatory nausea and vomiting.

Antiemetics given prior to chemotherapy can prevent nausea and vomiting in many patients. Certainly, relaxation, visual imagery, hypnosis, and other nonpharmacological measures have been helpful to these patients.

ALOPECIA

Hair loss is a common side effect of many chemotherapeutic agents. Although it is not life-threatening, alopecia can lower self-esteem and can serve as a reminder that the individual is undergoing treatment for his or her disease. Some patients find

Table 6-2

Emetogenic Potential of Chemotherapeutic Agents

Highly Emetogenic Agents Requiring Aggressive Antiemetic Therapy

- Carmustine (BCNU)
- Cisplatin
- Dacarbazine (DTIC)
- Streptozocin
- Dactinomycin
- Mechlorethamine

Moderately Emetogenic Agents

- Mithramycin
- Mitomycin
- Cytarabine
- Procarbazine
- Mitoxantrone
- Cyclophosphamide

Mildly Emetogenic Agents

- Vincristine
- Etoposide
- Vinblastine
- 5-Fluorouracil
- Bleomycin
- Methotrexate

Reprinted with permission from: Lind, J: Nursing Management of Nausea and Vomiting, Syllabus, Scripps Memorial Hospitals Ninth Cancer Symposium, 1989.

hair loss so disturbing that they refuse therapy because of it.

Once again, the nurse has a vital role in teaching and counseling the patient and the patient's family. If hair loss is unavoidable, patients may feel better about themselves if their appearance can be improved by wearing wigs, turbans, scarves, or hats. Remind patients that hair loss is almost always temporary and can be manifested by hair thinning or total hair loss. Alopecia occurs because of chemotherapy's effect on rapidly dividing cells. Often regrowth will begin even before chemotherapy ends. Some patients have noted that regrown hair is different from the hair they lost. It can be thicker, darker, curlier, or a slightly different color than it was before.

Not all drugs cause complete hair loss. The degree of alopecia depends on the specific drug, dosage, and method of administration. Drugs frequently associated with severe alopecia include doxorubicin, cyclophosphamide, and vinblastine. Drugs commonly associated with gradual thinning include methotrexate, 5FU, bleomycin, vincristine, and etoposide.

ANOREXIA AND WEIGHT LOSS

Weakness, loss of appetite, and general deterioration can develop as a patient's cancer progresses and treatments continue. Malnourished patients rarely can tolerate full doses of chemotherapy. Weight loss often results in reduced tolerance to chemotherapy and a less than optimal tumor response to the treatment.

Encourage patients who lose weight while receiving chemotherapy to eat foods (except red meats) that are high in protein. Many patients with advanced cancers have an aversion to red meat and foods high in carbohydrates. Nutritional supplements also may be prescribed and generally are tolerated.

It is not unusual for patients to complain of alterations in the sense of taste during the course of chemotherapy. Cyclophosphamide and vincristine are two drugs commonly associated with anorexia and changes in taste. Encourage patients to chew gum or to eat a tart candy during administration of the chemotherapy to help mask an unpleasant taste.

Warn patients beforehand that their appetitites may be poor during treatment and emphasize that maintaining nutrition is important even though it is difficult. Frequent small meals are often more appetizing than large meals, which can appear overwhelming. High-protein finger foods, such as cheese or peanut butter and crackers, can be appealing.

If a patient continues to lose weight, a feeding tube may be used to administer a nutritionally complete liquid diet. Although this is not an ideal feeding method, the patient who is malnourished and weak can benefit from such intervention.

CONSTIPATION

Constipation is a side effect of agents that affect the autonomic nervous system and its innervation of the bowel. Among agents causing constipation are vincristine and vinblastine. Usually constipation occurs after the drug has been given for a while. Older patients are more likely to experience constipation in general, and the addition of chemotherapy increases the likelihood. The best way to treat constipation is to prevent it. Have patients start the following before therapy begins:

- Increase fiber in the diet. (Increase fiber gradually; it may take at least a week before the increase has any effect on constipation.)
- Increase consumption of liquids (at least 8 glasses/day).
- Participate in light exercise regularly.
- Establish a calm, regular atmosphere for defecation.
- Take hot liquids when bowel stimulation is needed.
- Use bulk laxatives or stool softeners, when appropriate.

Assessment of the causes of constipation should include activity level, age, medication (i.e., narcotics, phenothiazines, diruetics, antihistamines, anticholinergics), depression, and long-term use of laxatives.

DIARRHEA

Diarrhea can be a side effect of chemotherapy, especially when the agent is an antimetabolite. When this problem occurs, therapy is delayed or stopped or the dose may be decreased. Thorough assessment of the cause of the diarrhea should determine its basis: the disease process itself, the treatment, impaction, or an overuse of laxatives. Measures to manage diarrhea include following a low-residue diet while the bowel rests. Monitor levels of electrolytes, and provide supplements as needed. Ensure adequate intake of fluids, and start IV hydration if necessary.

NEPHROTOXIC EFFECTS

Other aspects of compromised nerve innervation involve the kidney and bladder. Renal toxic effects can occur after administration of agents such as cisplatin, and methotrexate. If laboratory data suggest that nephrotoxic effects are occurring, chemotherapy may be delayed or discontinued. Depending on the agent, laboratory data used to monitor these effects include levels of blood urea nitrogen, creatinine, uric acid, protein, albumin, and electrolytes. Patients may have dysuria, an increase in the frequency or urgency of urination, or hematuria. Adequate hydration is the key to managing nephrotoxic effects, and aggressive hydration is part of the treatment if these effects do occur. Other procedures may be used also. For example, toxic levels of methotrexate cause precipitation of the drug in the renal tubules, and sodium bicarbonate can be given to alkalinize the urine.

SECONDARY MALIGNANCY

Unfortunately, chemotherapy may induce other malignancies. For example, leukemia or non-Hodgkin's lymphoma has developed in some patients treated for Hodgkin's disease. Bladder cancers have developed in patients treated with cyclophosphamide. Researchers think that the alterations in DNA caused by these agents may be the cause of these secondary malignancies. These alterations may be enhanced by radiation therapy.

GONADAL DYSFUNCTION

Testicular and ovarian function can be affected by many chemotherapeutic agents. Examples are the alkylating agents mechlorethamine and cyclophosphamide. The degree of dysfunction is worse if the patient also receives radiation therapy to the gonadal region.

In men, chemotherapy causes a depletion of the general epithelial lining of the seminiferous tubules. This can reduce or eliminate production of spermatocytes, resulting in oligospermia or azospermia. Infertility may be temporary or permanent, depending on the cumulative dosage and age of the patient. Although self-esteem and emotional well-being may be affected, sexual drive and physical capability usually are not impaired because of chemotherapy. Antifertility effects may be reversible in some cases after therapy has stopped. Reversal may be only partial, however, and it may take months or years to occur. If the proposed chemotherapy may cause sterility, men may wish to consider depositing some of their sperm in a sperm bank before they begin chemotherapy.

In women, amenorrhea can occur with most chemotherapeutic agents. The degree of ovarian failure is strongly related to the age of the patient and the cumulative dose of the drugs. In some patients, menstruation may resume. Women more than 30 years old have the highest prevalence of ovarian failure. Women can have signs and symptoms of menopause, including amenorrhea, hot flashes, insomnia, irritability, dyspareunia, and vaginal dryness. Estrogen replacement therapy may be helpful.

No evidence exists demonstrating increased chromosomal abnormalities or congenital abnormalities in the offspring of persons who have received chemotherapy. The prevalence of spontaneous abortion in women who have had chemotherapy is no higher than that of women in the general population. However, pregnancies in women with a history of chemotherapy should be monitored more carefully for residual chemotherapeutic effects and for congenital abnormalities in the fetus.

EXTRAVASATION

Some chemotherapeutic agents are called vesicants because they can damage or destroy local tissue when they leak into that tissue around the administration site. Examples of such agents are doxorubicin, mitomycin, and vincristine.

Efforts to prevent extravasation are crucial when administering vesicant agents. If these agents infiltrate into surrounding tissue during IV administration, they can destroy the tissue and ultimately leave the area necrotic and, when affected ligaments are involved, nonfunctional. If extravasation occurs, notify the physician immediately.

Guidelines to prevent extravasation have been published by various professional organizations. The following lists major principles in the prevention and treatment of extravasation adopted by the Oncology Nursing Society. For detailed information about these recommendations, read them in their entirety.

1. Continually monitor patients who receive vesicants during and after administration.

2. Prevention of extravasation is the priority in dealing with agents that are vesicants. (See Table 6-3.) To prevent extravasation, follow safe, thorough technique for IV access. Slowly infuse the drug, and flush the line frequently. Be sure that IV access is good and that blood return is adequate (although blood return is not always a guarantee that the site is good). Check the site by aspirating a few milliliters of fluid every few minutes. Be sure the site is stabilized properly during administration. Discontinue the infusion if the patient states he or she is uncomfortable. The order of infusing vesicants (in combination regimens) remains controversial.

3. Have antidotes or equipment readily available so that any extravasation can be treated immediately.

4. If extravasation occurs, stop the administration of the drug. Keep the needle in place so that residual drug can be aspirated from the site. Then administer the antidote (clockwise SC around the site with a small-gauge needle). If recommended, apply warm or cool compresses to the site and/or elevate the arm (if a peripheral site). Do not apply pressure to the site. Cover the site with an occlusive, sterile dressing.

Table 6-3
Vesicant and Irritant Antineoplastic Drugs

Vesicant Drugs	Irritant Drugs
Dactinomycin (Cosmegan®)	Carmustine (BiCNU®)
Daunorubicin (Cerubidine®)	Dacarbazine (DTIC-Dome®)
Doxorubicin (Adriamycin®)	Etoposide (Vepesid®)
Mechlorethamine (nitrogen mustard)	Plicamycin (Mithracin®)
Vinblastine sulfate (Velban®)	Streptozocin (Zanosar®)
Vincristine (Oncovin®)	Teniposide (Vumon®)
Vinorelbinel (Navelbine®)	

Carter, P., Engelking, C., Finstuen, K., et al. (1988). *Cancer chemotherapy: Guidelines,* Modules I-V (Module V, p. 7). Pittsburgh: Oncology Nursing Society. Reprinted with permission.

5. Observe the site on an ongoing basis, and note any increases in pain, redness, or swelling.

6. Document the extravasation and its treatment. Include a photograph of the site, the date, time, size and type of needle, a description of the site, amount and name of drug administered, management measures taken, patient's complaints, and notification of the physician.

A sample extravasation record is shown in Figure 6-1.

ANAPHYLAXIS

Some agents are known to cause an anaphylactic or allergic response in some patients. Examples of these agents are bleomycin and L-asparaginase. The following reviews guidelines, published by the Oncology Nursing Society, for nurses who administer such agents. Before giving these agents, refer to these recommendations and/or manufacturers' guidelines.

1. Continually monitor patients who receive agents that might cause an allergic reaction. Be sure the patient's record includes a history of any allergies.

2. Prevention of an allergic reaction is the priority in dealing with these agents. If warranted, give a test dose of the agent or do a skin test before giving the regular dose. Observe the patient for at least 15 minutes before giving the regular dose.

3. Have antidotes or equipment readily available so that any anaphylactic reaction can be treated immediately.

4. Administer the agent slowly, and observe the patient for at least 15 minutes after administration.

5. If a reaction occurs (either local or systemic), stop administration of the drug. Maintain IV access and hydrate if appropriate. If warranted, administer an antidote. Make sure the patient is positioned so that vital organs can be perfused. Take vital signs frequently. Maintain the airway.

6. Observe the patient and/or site on an ongoing basis. Signs and symptoms of a systemic aller-

gic reaction include respiratory arrest, wheezing, itching, chest tightness, agitation, dizziness, nausea, cramping, chills, and hypotension. A localized reaction might include urticaria, wheals, and swelling.

7. Document the allergic reaction. Include the name of the drug administered and the amount, management measures taken, the patient's complaints, and notification of the physician.

Figure 6-1

Extravasation Record

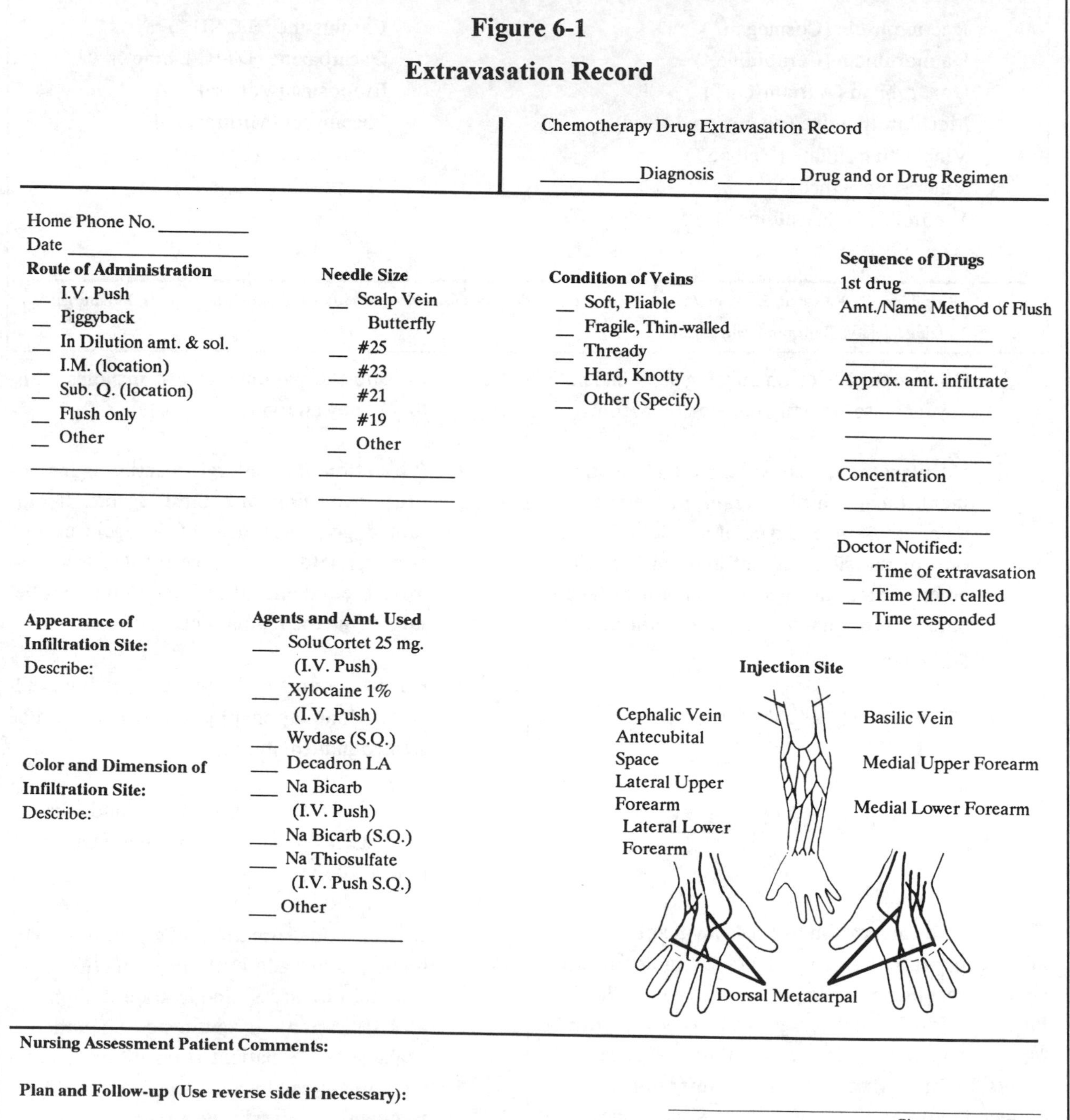

Chemotherapy Drug Extravasation Record

__________Diagnosis _________Drug and or Drug Regimen

Home Phone No. __________

Date _______________

Route of Administration

- __ I.V. Push
- __ Piggyback
- __ In Dilution amt. & sol.
- __ I.M. (location)
- __ Sub. Q. (location)
- __ Flush only
- __ Other

Needle Size

- __ Scalp Vein Butterfly
- __ #25
- __ #23
- __ #21
- __ #19
- __ Other

Condition of Veins

- __ Soft, Pliable
- __ Fragile, Thin-walled
- __ Thready
- __ Hard, Knotty
- __ Other (Specify)

Sequence of Drugs

1st drug ______

Amt./Name Method of Flush

Approx. amt. infiltrate

Concentration

Doctor Notified:

- __ Time of extravasation
- __ Time M.D. called
- __ Time responded

Appearance of Infiltration Site:
Describe:

Color and Dimension of Infiltration Site:
Describe:

Agents and Amt. Used

- ___ SoluCortet 25 mg. (I.V. Push)
- ___ Xylocaine 1% (I.V. Push)
- ___ Wydase (S.Q.)
- ___ Decadron LA
- ___ Na Bicarb (I.V. Push)
- ___ Na Bicarb (S.Q.)
- ___ Na Thiosulfate (I.V. Push S.Q.)
- ___ Other

Injection Site

Nursing Assessment Patient Comments:

Plan and Follow-up (Use reverse side if necessary):

Signature and Date

Created by Lcdr Judith Ann Killman, BSN, MA, MS., 1990.

PAIN

Patients with cancer can suffer because of the disease itself rather than the treatment. Chemotherapy in general does not cause pain, but some treatments contribute to patients' reports of pain.

When patients are treated with chemotherapy, common pain syndromes may occur. Peripheral neuropathy, associated with vinca alkaloids, is reported first as a tingling in the extremities that occurs after administration of the chemotherapeutic agent. The pain can advance to a chronic condition, when patients have unrelenting aching and tingling with some numbness. Symptoms are muscle and joint tenderness when touched and diffuse myalgias. This pain can subside when steroid treatments begin again or when treatment is stopped gradually.

PSYCHOSOCIAL CONCERNS

Much attention in recent years has been devoted to the pivotal influence of a patient's support system and the emphasis that needs to be placed on the patient's ability to cope with whatever resources available. Management of the psychosocial aspects of cancer treatment requires adequate teaching to address knowledge deficits of the patient and the patient's family. Research suggests that patients who have information about what is happening to them and have tools to make decisions comply with treatment better and maintain some control and influence over the outcome of their therapy.

A patient's ability to cope with the stress associated with treatment is affected by social supports and the patient's ability to adapt. Certainly, management of the side effects of chemotherapy relies on patients who can mobilize those forces. The goal of treatment is to maintain functioning and quality of life. In order to reach that goal, patients need to have information, need to express and boost their feeling of self-worth and independence, and need to show they can cope, by maintaning cognitive processes and positive behavior. Managing the period of chemotherapy cannot be accomplished without addressing these psychosocial concerns (Barsevick, & McCarthy, 1990).

EXAM QUESTIONS

Chapter 6

Questions 46–68

46. How does chemotherapy cause thrombocytopenia?

  a. It decreases the production of platelets in the bone marrow.
  b. It alters the clotting factors.
  c. It increases circulating platelets.
  d. It increases the number of granulocytes.

47. A high risk of spontaneous hemorrhage is most likely to occur if the platelet count is less than

  a. 75,000 cells/cu mm
  b. 20,000 cells/cu mm
  c. 250,000 cells/cu mm
  d. 1,000,000 cells/cu mm

48. Chemotherapy may increase the risk of infection by which of the following mechanisms?

  a. Repairing the integrity of skin and mucous membranes
  b. Increasing nutritional status
  c. Suppressing the white blood cells in the bone marrow
  d. Lowering levels of antibiotic in the bloodstream

49. One of the causes of nausea or vomiting in patients receiving chemotherapy is

  a. Fatigue
  b. Stimulation of the chemoreceptor trigger zone
  c. Hyperthermia
  d. Overhydration

50. Chemotherapeutic agents that have a severe emetic action include

  a. Bleomycin and 5FU
  b. Cisplatin and carmustine
  c. Vincristine and L-asparaginase
  d. Carmustine and prednisone

51. Grade II stomatitis is defined as

  a. Reddening
  b. White patches over 15% of oral mucosa
  c. Small patches of ulceration
  d. Ulcerations and bleeding

52. Which of the following statements about alopecia as a side effect of chemotherapy is correct?

  a. It occurs because chemotherapy attacks slowly dividing cells.
  b. It can be treated with antiemetics.
  c. It can be manifested either as hair thinning or as total hair loss.
  d. It is never a disturbing side effect.

53. Interventions that prevent or minimize extravasation of chemotherapeutic agents include

  a. Monitoring the patient throughout administration
  b. Infusing the agent rapidly and flushing the vein frequently with normal saline
  c. Ensuring the patency of the vein by assessing for an adequate blood return 30 minutes after administration of the agent
  d. Giving the infusion at 1-hour intervals if discomfort at the infusion site is noted

54. Which of the following statements about bleomycin is correct?

    a. It should be prepared 2 days before administration.
    b. It is orange.
    c. It requires ample antiemetic coverage.
    d. It can cause allergic reactions.

55. How should vesicants be administered?

    a. As rapidly as possible
    b. With caution to avoid extravasation
    c. Directly into an artery
    d. Into the feet

56. Vesicant chemotherapeutic agents include

    a. 5FU etoposide, streptozocin
    b. Dactinomycin, doxorubicin dacarbazine
    c. Carmustine, cisplatin, vinblastine
    d. Daunorubicin, mechlorethamine, vinblastine

57. The best way to manage extravasation is to

    a. Use veins that are hard and sclerosed.
    b. Prevent it from happening.
    c. Infuse the agent rapidly.
    d. Make sure the physician gives the agent.

58. What side effect is caused by most chemotherapeutic agents?

    a. Myelosuppression
    b. Increase in WBC count
    c. Bradycardia
    d. Increased appetite

59. How long is the life span of a leukocyte?

    a. 6 hours
    b. 6 days
    c. 12 hours
    d. 12 days

60. How long after administration of vinblastine does recovery of the WBC count occur?

    a. 3–5 days
    b. 14–21 days
    c. 7 days
    d. 8–12 days

61. A good indicator of a patient's actual ability to fight infection is the

    a. Absolute granulocyte count
    b. WBC count
    c. Platelet count
    d. Hemoglobin level

62. Patients receiving a drug known to decrease the number of platelets should be instructed to report which of the following findings immediately?

    a. Shortness of breath
    b. Fever
    c. Change of hair color
    d. Increased bruising

63. Stomatitis generally occurs how many days after chemotherapy?

    a. 2–4
    b. 3–6
    c. 5–7
    d. 8–12

64. Patients receiving chemotherapy should be encouraged to eat which of the following?

    a. Foods high in protein and carbohydrates
    b. Red meat
    c. Fatty foods
    d. Spicy foods

65. Constipation can occur in the patient receiving which of the following chemotherapeutic agents?

    a. 5FU
    b. Vincristine
    c. Methotrexate
    d. ARA-C

66. Treatment of which cancer has been associated with secondary malignancies?

    a. Melanoma
    b. Hodgkin's disease
    c. Giloblastomas
    d. Lung cancer

67. Sperm banking may be considered for male patients receiving which of the following?

    a. Mycostatin
    b. Alkylating agents
    c. Antibiotics
    d. Blood transfusions

68. Two drugs that may cause anaphylaxis are

    a. Cytoxan and bleomycin
    b. Vincristine and vinblastine
    c. Bleomycin and L-asparaginase
    d. Nitrogen mustard and 5FU

CHAPTER 7

DEVELOPMENTS IN CHEMOTHERAPY

CHAPTER OBJECTIVE

After completing this chapter, you will be able to describe additional approaches to chemotherapy.

LEARNING OBJECTIVES

After reading this chapter, you will be able to

1. Identify three acronyms for combination chemotherapy.
2. Describe how chemotherapy functions when it is prescribed with surgery or radiation therapy.
3. Specify three tasks of the nurse who is giving chemotherapy as part of a clinical trial.

Chemotherapy as a treatment for cancer continues to develop in certain directions. Among these are the following:

- More use of chemotherapeutic agents in combination with one another or with another treatment, such as surgery, radiation, or immunotherapy
- Development of new drugs or analogues of existing drugs, which have fewer side effects
- Increased or aggressive dosages to attain the best response for cure or best control
- Adjuvant chemotherapy, which boosts initial surgical or radiation treatments, to eliminate remaining cancer cells or metastases
- Development of growth factors, which make it possible to use aggressive dosages of the chemotherapeutic agent and still spare the bone marrow or support its growth or maintenance
- Use of potentiators with chemotherapy
- Chemotherapy as a source of prevention for cancer

COMBINATION CHEMOTHERAPY

Using more than one chemotherapeutic agent for the treatment of cancer is not a new approach. Adding agents to a course of chemotherapy increases the action on tumor cells during the cell cycle. Using more than one agent also can diversify the side effects that any one agent might cause alone. For example, Figure 7-1 shows the nadirs associated with MOPP or ABVD (see the following for explanation of the acronyms). Clearly, identical nadirs for all these drugs have been avoided by scheduling administration of these agents appropriately. Additionally, in some cases, a patient who has become resistant to one agent might respond to the synergistic action or accumulation of multiple agents against the tumor.

Examples of chemotherapy given in combination abound. The acronyms for the agents used have become the names of the therapy. One of the oldest effective combination chemotherapies is MOPP. MOPP refers to a regimen of mechlorethamine or nitrogen mustard (M), vincristine or Oncovin (O),

Figure 7-1

MOPP/ABVD Administration Schedule and Corresponding White Blood Cell Count Nadirs

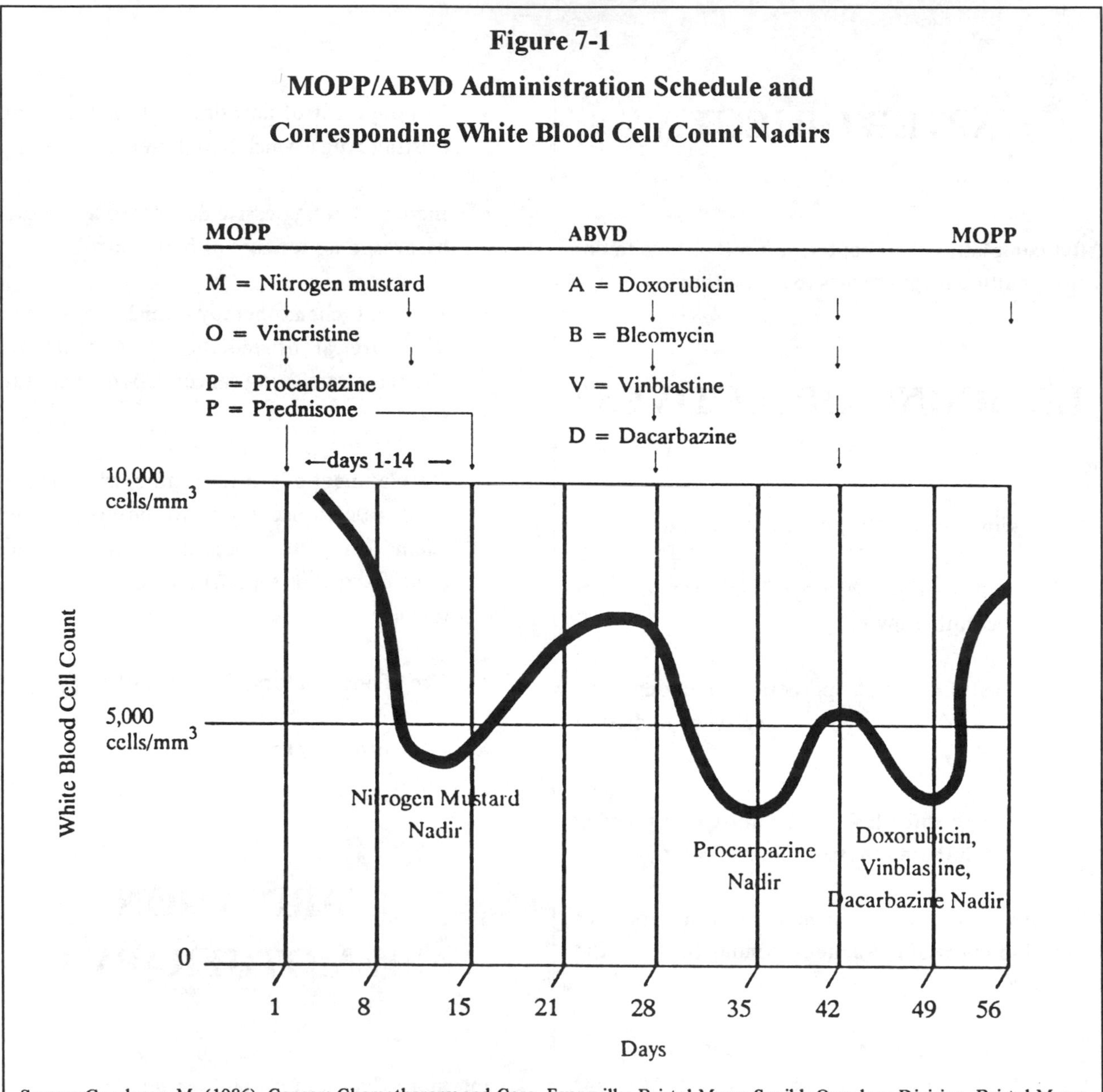

Source: Goodman, M. (1986). Cancer: Chemotherapy and Care. Evansville: Bristol-Myers Squibb Oncology Division, Bristol-Myers Squibb Company. Reprinted with permission.

procarbazine (P), and prednisone (P). MOPP has been used for more than 25 years as a treatment for Hodgkin's disease, when it is treated in the late stages of development. A standard regimen of MOPP is as follows:

- Mechlorethamine: 6 mg/m^2 IV on Days 1 and 8
- Vincristine (Oncovin): 1.4 mg/m^2 IV on Days 1 and 8 (maximum of 2 mg)
- Procarbazine: 100 mg/m^2 orally on Days 1–14
- Prednisone: 40 mg/m^2 orally on Days 1–14, cycles 1 and 4 only.

Cycles of MOPP would be repeated every 28 days. Patients first treated with MOPP have had impressive complete response (80%) and survival rates (68%) two decades after therapy.

Table 7-1 lists some of the more standard combination chemotherapy regimens that will be refined or changed in time as treatment approaches.

Chemotherapy also is being used more in combination with other modes of treatment, such as radiation or surgery. This is referred to as combined modality therapy. Chemotherapy is used to reduce the tumor burden before surgery, so the surgeon can attempt to remove most if not all of the tumor. Chemotherapy used in this way is sometimes called neoadjuvant chemotherapy. Studies are under way on the use of chemotherapy in combination with other therapies in the treatment of colonic, pancreatic, and lung cancers.

Administration of selected chemotherapeutic agents before radiation therapy can increase the sensitivity of tumor cells to radiation. This approach is used in treating non-small-cell lung cancer in its later but still treatable stages. Cisplatin and fluorouracil, for example, are given before or at the same time as radiation therapy. Moreover, if the tumor shrinks enough, the surgeon can choose to resect what has become a smaller mass.

Immunotherapy, the most recent mode of treatment, attempts to boost or recreate the body's defenses to thwart foreign invasion or infection. Even though immunotherapeutic agents can be given via the same routes of administration as chemotherapeutic agents, most of these agents are not specifically cytotoxic. Instead, modifying the biological response, immunotherapy makes the environment inhospitable to the tumor or activates the body's cells, which can kill or suppress tumor cells. The combination of chemotherapy and immunotherapy can be more effective than either one alone.

For example, when used in tandem with chemotherapy, interferon (a biological response modifier) can increase the number of cells killed in leukemias and lymphomas. Other uses of immunotherapy to potentiate chemotherapy involves the use of interferon in treatments of renal cancer.

NEW DRUGS

More effective, less toxic drugs are always in development, although additions to the current arsenal of chemotherapeutic agents has slowed since the 1970s. Efforts to improve on the agents already used have focused on analogues or variations of those drugs. An example of this is carboplatin (Paraplatin), an analogue of cisplatin. Carboplatin is less toxic than cisplatin to the kidneys and inner ear, but can be equal in its effectiveness in regimens that use cisplatin. In some cases, patients have reported less nausea and vomiting with carboplatin.

Another approach has been the development of couplers for established agents, which can minimize some of the main, dose-limiting side effects of the agent. An example is mesna (Mesnex), an agent that can help prevent hemorrhagic cystitis caused by a recently developed analogue of cyclophosphamide, ifosfamide.

Table 7-1
Combination Chemotherapies

Type of Cancer Treated	Acronym	Drugs Used
Breast cancer	CAF	Cyclophosphamide Doxorubicin (Adriamycin) Fluorouracil (5FU)
	CMF	Cyclophosphamide Methotrexate Fluorouracil (5FU)
Colonic cancer	F-CL	Fluorouracil (5FU) Calcium leucovorin
Genitourinary cancer	CAP	Cisplatin Doxorubicin (Adriamycin) Cyclophosphamide
Head and neck cancer	CF	Cisplatin Fluorouracil (5FU)
Leukemias		
Acute myelogenous, induction	COAP	Cyclophosphamide Vincristine (Oncovin) Cytarabine (ARA-C) Prednisone
Lymphoma		
Hodgkin	ABVD	Doxorubicin (Adriamycin) Bleomycin Vinblastine Dacarbazine
Non-Hodgkin	CHOP	Cyclophosphamide Doxorubicin (Adriamycin) Vincristine (Oncovin) Prednisone
Ovarian cancer	AP	Doxorubicin (Adriamycin) Cisplatin
	CDC	Carboplatin Doxorubicin (Adriamycin) Cyclophosphamide
Cancer in children Acute lymphocytic leukemia, induction	DVP	Daunorubicin Vincristine Prednisone
Testicular cancer	PEB	Platinum Etoposide Bleomycin

Created by Ellen Carr, RN, MSN, 1990.

Ifosfamide, an analog of cyclophosphamide, has been approved as a third-line treatment for testicular cancer (the therapy usually includes cisplatin and etoposide). Ifosfamide is not to be given without mesna. Before this coupler for ifosfamide was established, ifosfamide itself was too toxic an agent to use effectively.

DOSAGES

Studies repeatedly show that standard dosages or aggressive approaches to treatment have cured cancer or enabled periods of sustained control of the disease. Reduced dosages and elimination of some of the courses of therapy once were championed as ways to provide more tolerable treatments for patients. However, these changes were not beneficial, as disease would recur quickly or sustained remissions were not achievable.

Now clinicians advocate using the largest dose that can be tolerated. An example of this approach can be found in cisplatin regimens. Now more concentrated efforts are made to control the disturbing side effect of nausea and vomiting rather than reduce the dose of cisplatin. Therefore, more effective antiemetic regimens, which include pharmacological, psychological, and combination approaches make it possible to use high doses of cisplatin.

ADJUVANT CHEMOTHERAPY

As discussed in previous chapters, adjuvant chemotherapy is the addition of chemotherapy courses after other treatment modes, such as surgery or radiation. These courses attempt to eliminate remaining tumor cells or prevent metastases.

Advances in adjuvant treatment have paralelled improvements in the imaging and staging of tumors on the molecular and cellular level. Still, ways to detect the spread of a tumor are limited, and ways to provide some early assurance that local disease has not spread remain elusive. The necessity for adjuvant chemotherapy is being debated regularly in the medical community. Two of the most prominent cancers treated with an adjuvant approach are breast and colonic cancers.

As an example, adjuvant treatment for a classification of colonic cancer (Duke's stage C) has included courses of 5FU and levamisole. After this type of tumor has been removed by the surgeon, chemotherapy is used in an attempt to kill or prevent the spread of any residual tumor undetected by diagnostic equipment currently available.

COLONY STIMULATING FACTORS (CSFs)

CSFs have been developed to support or stimulate cells produced by the bone marrow. Most chemotherapies cause what seems to be the universal side effect: bone marrow suppression. These growth factors attempt to quicken the recovery of granulocytes and monocytes, so that patients can receive maximal doses of chemotherapeutic agents and be at less risk for infection or other complications associated with myelosuppression.

These agents have names that specify the cell lines they support or regulate: granulocyte/macrophage colony-stimulating factor (GM-CSF), granulocyte colony-stimulating factor (G-CSF), and macrophage colony-stimulating factor (M-CSF). In addition to accelerating the recovery of bone marrow cells, growth factors can reverse bone marrow suppression. Because these factors also may stimulate development of malignant cells (i.e., leukemias), studies are concentrating on targeting these agents and timing their delivery to optimize chemotherapy cell kill.

For patients with chronic anemia from their disease or chemotherapy, erythropoietin is also available. This hormone stimulates the production of red blood cells; the intent is to thwart the anemia and reduce the need for blood transfusions.

PREVENTION

Strategies to prevent cancers have included chemotherapy of sorts. In animal tests, synthetic retinoids (specifically, vitamin A) have reduced cervical, squamous cell, colonic, and lung cancers. Unfortunately, vitamin A is too toxic to be practical, at this point, as a treatment. Still, work continues to determine if this might be a way to prevent recurrence of cancer or to reduce the prevalence of cancer in high-risk groups.

CLINICAL TRIALS

Studies of new drugs are ongoing. Research progresses to animal models and then to trials in humans. The National Cancer Institute (NCI) is a major sponsor of new drug trials. Its criteria allows for one in four drugs presented to be included in initial drug trials. (The pool of drugs submitted to the NCI totals about 40,000 drugs a year.) The sifting process continues to determine the better drugs to try on humans. Only about 10 drugs are actually chosen as worthy for clinical use. Those drugs go through schedules to determine appropriate routes and expected toxic effects. Only after that is completed can clinical trials on humans begin.

Studies are broken down into three distinct phases:

1. Phase I: Defines toxicities and maximum tolerated dose. Investigates pharmacology.

2. Phase II: Determines antitumor activity and side effects at a given dose and schedule.

3. Phase III: Compares the therapy under study with other therapies.

Chemotherapeutic agents that already have been tested in clinical trials can be tested again for different tumors at different stages of growth. As mentioned earlier, chemotherapy used in conjunction with other methods of treatment also should go through the clinical-trial process. Therefore, nurses who are not certified to give chemotherapy frequently may care for patients who are enrolled in these trials. Efforts continue to expand clinical trials away from major research centers. Eligible patients are being recruited from a much wider population pool, including community hospitals, private physicians' offices, and rural cancer treatment networks.

A nurse who provides care for patients in clinical trials needs to make sure that written informed consent has been obtained and that patients understand aspects of their participation in the study. The nurse serves as one of the main observers of the patient, the patient advocate, master interpreter, and integral data collector when patients are receiving these drugs. This responsibility is just as important as that of administering the drug. Chemotherapy cannot progress without the nurse who looks at overall therapy options for the patient.

DELIVERY OPTIONS: CHEMOTHERAPY ADMINISTRATION AWAY FROM THE HOSPITAL

As cost-cutting measures continue to be predominate in health care delivery, the environment in which chemotherapy is administered will change. The trend to deliver chemotherapy on an outpatient basis or in the home will continue to flourish. Technology, in the form of ambulatory infusion devices, unit dose drug delivery systems, long-term catheters, and sophisticated monitoring devices is propelling this push out of a standard hospital for treatment. These products and services can only expand as chemotherapeutic treatments advance. Expert nursing care to support and monitor this delivery approach will continue to be a highly sought after commodity.

EXAM QUESTIONS

Chapter 7

Questions 69–75

69. What is adjuvant chemotherapy?

    a. Courses of chemotherapy given after other modes of treatment to destroy remaining cancer cells and prevent metastases
    b. Surgery and radiation therapy given together
    c. Two or more chemotherapeutic agents given concurrently
    d. Chemotherapy given to reduce a large tumor burden

70. Which of the following is an example of combination chemotherapy?

    a. MOPP
    b. Surgery and cisplatin
    c. Radiation and 5FU
    d. Vincristine and vitamins

71. MOPP, a combination chemotherapy used in advanced Hodgkin's disease, includes which drugs?

    a. Doxorubicin, prednisone, cisplatin, nitrogen mustard
    b. Nitrogen mustard, vincristine, procarbazine, prednisone
    c. Bleomycin, vinblastine, dacarbazine, methotrexate
    d. Cytoxan, nitrogen mustard, bleomycin, BCNU

72. What is tested during phase II clinical trials for new drug therapies?

    a. Toxic levels
    b. Side effects
    c. Comparison therapies
    d. Maximal tolerated dose

73. What is the role of growth factors in cancer treatment?

    a. They allow chemotherapeutic molecules to grow.
    b. They allow quick recovery of granuloytes and platelets.
    c. They are attacked by chemotherapeutic agents because they are tumors.
    d. They change the hormonal environment.

74. A common combination for chemotherapy is

    a. ZZN
    b. LQR
    c. CHOP
    d. MRI

75. A growth factor that stimulates production of red blood cells is

    a. GM-CSF
    b. Erythropoietin
    c. G-CSF
    d. MOPP

BIBLIOGRAPHY

Barsevick, A., & McCarthy, P. (1990). The treatment/chronicity phase. In S. Groenwald, et al. *Cancer nursing principles and practice* (2nd ed., pp. 114–121). Boston: Jones and Barlett.

Belinson, J. L. (1980). Understanding how cancer chemotherapy works. *Contemporary OB/GYN 21*, 2–17.

Bender, C. (1987). *Chemotherapy: Core curriculum for oncology nursing* (p. 228). Philadelphia: Saunders.

Brown, A. E. (1985). Neutropenia, fever, and infection. In A. E. Brown & D. Armstrong (Eds.). *Infectious complications of neoplastic disease: Controversies in management (pp. 19–34). New Y*ork: Yorke Medical Books.

Burnett, P. (1982). *Model inservice curriculum for oncology nursing.* American Cancer Society, California Division.

Carter, P., Engelking, C., Finstuen, K., et al. (1988). *Cancer chemotherapy: Guidelines*, Modules I-V (Module V, p. 7). Pittsburgh: Oncology Nursing Society.

Casciato, L. & Lowitz, B. B. (1983). *Manual of bedside oncology.* Boston: Little, Brown and Company.

Chapman, R. M. (1984). Effect of cytotoxic therapy on sexuality and gonadal function (pp. 343–351). In M. C. Parry & J. W. Yarbro (Eds.). *Toxicity of chemotherapy.* New York: Grune & Stratton.

Cloak, M. M., Connor, T. H., Stevens, K. R., et al. (1985). Occupational exposure of nursing personnel to antineoplastic agents. *Oncology Nursing Forum, 12,* 33–39.

Dorr, R. T., & VonHoff D. D. (1994). Cancer Chemotherapy Handbook, 2nd edition, Norwalk, CT: Appleton and Lange.

Goodman, M. (1986). *Cancer: Chemotherapy and care* (pp. 1–36). Evansville: Bristol-Myers Oncology Division, Bristol-Myers Co.

Goodman, M. S., & Wickham, R. (1984). Venous access devices: An overview. *Oncology Nursing Forum, 11,* 16–23.

Knobf, M. K., et al. (1984). *Cancer chemotherapy: Treatment and care.* Boston: G. K. Hall Medical.

Lind, J. (1989). *Nursing Management of Nausea and Vomiting* (Syllabus). Scripps Memorial Hospitals Ninth Cancer Symposium.

Longman, A. (1990). Cancer nursing education. In S. Groenwald, et al. *Cancer nursing principles and practice* (2nd ed., pp. 815–824). Boston: Jones and Barlett.

Meadows, A. T., & Silber, J. (1985). Delayed consequences of therapy for childhood cancer. *Cancer, 35,* 271-285.

Nursing 88 Drug Handbook (1988). (pp. 590–624). Springhouse, PA: Springhouse Corp.

Occupational Safety and Health Administration. (1986). *Guidelines for cytotoxic antineoplastic drugs.* Washington, DC: U.S. Department of Labor.

Occupational Safety and Health Administration. (January 1986). Instruction Publication 8-1.1. Washington, DC: U.S. Department of Labor.

Occupational Safety and Health Administration. (December, 1991). The Federal Register, Volume 56, No. 235.

Oncology Nursing Society. (1984). *Cancer chemotherapy: Guidelines and recommendations for nursing education and practice* (pp. 1–19). Pittsburgh.

Perry, M. C. (1992). *The Chemotherapy Sourcebook.* Baltimore, MD: Williams and Wilkens.

Pitot, H. C. (1981). *Fundamentals of oncology* (2nd ed., pp. 1–119). New York: Marcel Dekker.

Reed, W. P., Newman, K. A., deJongh, C., et al. (1983). Prolonged venous access for chemotherapy by means of the Hickman catheter. *Cancer, 52,* 185–192.

Samson, M., Revkin, S., Jones, S., et al. (1984). Dose response and dose survival advantage for high vs. low dose cisplatinum combined with vinblastine and bleomycin in disseminated testicular cancer. Southwest Oncology Group Study. *Cancer, 53,* 1029–1035.

Skeel, R. T. (1982). The biologic and pharmacologic basis of cancer chemotherapy. In R. T. Skeel (Ed.). *Manual of cancer chemotherapy.* (pp. 3–12). Boston: Little, Brown.

Tenenbaum, L. (1989). *Cancer chemotherapy: A reference guide* (pp. 271–302). Philadelphia: Saunders.

Tenenbaum, L. (1987). Nursing administration of chemotherapy. *Chemotherapy: Core curriculum for oncology nursing* (p. 333). Philadelphia: Saunders.

Yarbro, C. H., & Perry, M. C. (1985). The effect of cancer therapy on gonadal function. *Seminars in Oncology Nursing, 1,* 3–8.

SUGGESTED READING LIST

DiVita, V. T., Hellman, S., & Rosenberg, S. A. (Eds.). (1993). *Cancer: Principles and practice of oncology* (4th ed.). Philadelphia: Lippincott.

Groenwald, S., et al. (1987). *Cancer nursing principles and practice* (2nd ed.). Boston: Jones and Bartlett.

Knobf, M. K., et al. (1984). *Cancer chemotherapy: Treatment and care.* Boston: G. K. Hall Medical.

McNally, J. C., et al. (Eds.). (1985). *Guidelines for cancer nursing practice.* Orlando, FL: Grune & Stratton.

Occupational Safety and Health Administration. (1986). *Guidelines for cytotoxic antineoplastic drugs.* Washington, DC: U.S. Department of Labor.

Oncology Nursing Society. (1988). *Cancer chemotherapy guidelines*, Modules I-V. Pittsburgh:

Tenenbaum, L. (1989). *Cancer chemotherapy: A reference guide.* Philadelphia: Saunders .

Ziegfeld, C. R. (Ed.). (1987). *Core curriculum for oncology nursing.* Philadelphia: Saunders.

GLOSSARY

adjuvant chemotherapy: chemotherapy after initial surgery or radiation treatment to destroy remaining cancer cells and prevent metastases.

alkylating agent: a chemotherapeutic agent that causes alkylation by binding to DNA and preventing its replication.

antiemetic: a drug that alleviates or stops nausea and/or vomiting.

antimetabolites: chemotherapeutic agent that substitutes for nucleotides in the DNA helix and prevents DNA synthesis.

antitumor antibiotic: chemotherapeutic agent that blocks DNA and RNA transcription. The action is similar to that of alkylating agents.

alopecia: loss of hair in which the hair follicle remains intact.

benign: growth that is not malignant.

carcinogen: an agent that causes cancer.

cell cycle: the stages of growth that a cell goes through: periods of DNA, RNA, and protein synthesis and transcription that lead to a period of cell division, creating two identical daughter cells during mitosis.

combination chemotherapy: the use of more than one chemotherapeutic agent to achieve better tumor cell kill and/or fewer or less severe side effects.

cytotoxic agent: drug used to kill cancer cells.

extravasation: discharge or escape of blood or fluid from a vessel into the tissues around the vessel, resulting in tissue necrosis and/or ulceration.

growth factors: factors that stimulate an increase in neutrophils; used to boost the compromised defenses against infection in neutropenic patients.

growth fraction: that portion of cells in a cell population that is dividing.

irritant: an agent that causes local inflammation and discomfort.

malignant: growth that cannot be controlled.

metastasize: spread of cancer cells to neighboring or distant organs or tissues.

nadir: the low point. In myelosuppression, the time when cell counts are lowest and suppression is maximal.

neoplasm: cancer cells; tumor.

neutropenia: a reduction in the number of neutrophils available to fight off bacteria or other sources of infection in the body.

nitrosourea: a lipid-soluble agent that blocks DNA synthesis in the cell.

palliation: treatment of signs and symptoms that provides relief but does not cure.

stomatitis: an inflammation of the rapidly dividing cells in the oral mucosa.

tumor: a collection of cancer cells.

tumor doubling time: the amount of time it takes a tumor to double in size.

thrombocytopenia: a decrease in the number of platelets.

Valsalva maneuver: forcible exhalation against the glottis, increasing intrathoracic pressure and impeding venous return to the heart.

vesicant: an agent that can cause blistering, resulting in cellular damage or tissue destruction.

vinca alkaloids: chemotherapeutic agents that halt mitosis by binding to the microtubules, blocking DNA strands so the cell cannot divide.

APPENDIX A

VENOUS ACCESS DEVICES

VASCULAR ACCESS DEVICES (VADs)

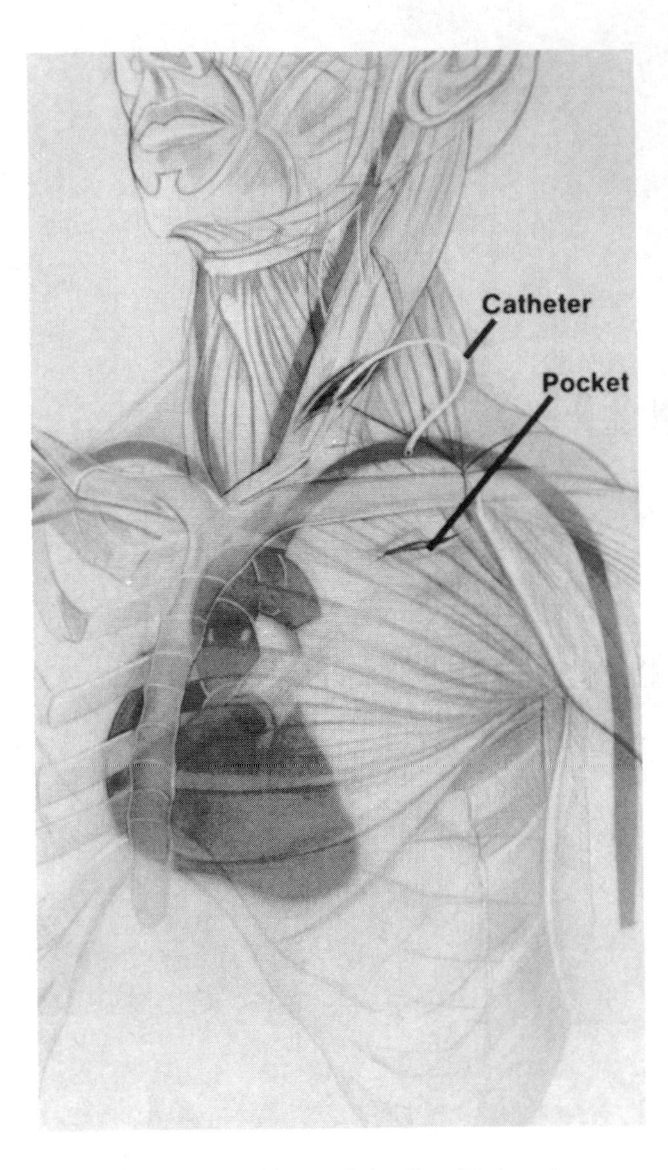

Drawing reprinted with permission from Pharmacia Deltec, Inc., St. Paul, MN.

Vascular access devices (VADs) provide a means of access for long-term medication or hydration therapy. Although these devices can provide direct access to an organ or particular region of the body, typically VADs are catheters leading to the heart. Long-term central venous access devices are surgically placed with their tip in the superior vena cava or the right atrium. This diagram shows the anatomical placement of a long-term central VAD. The following pages show a few examples of VADs.

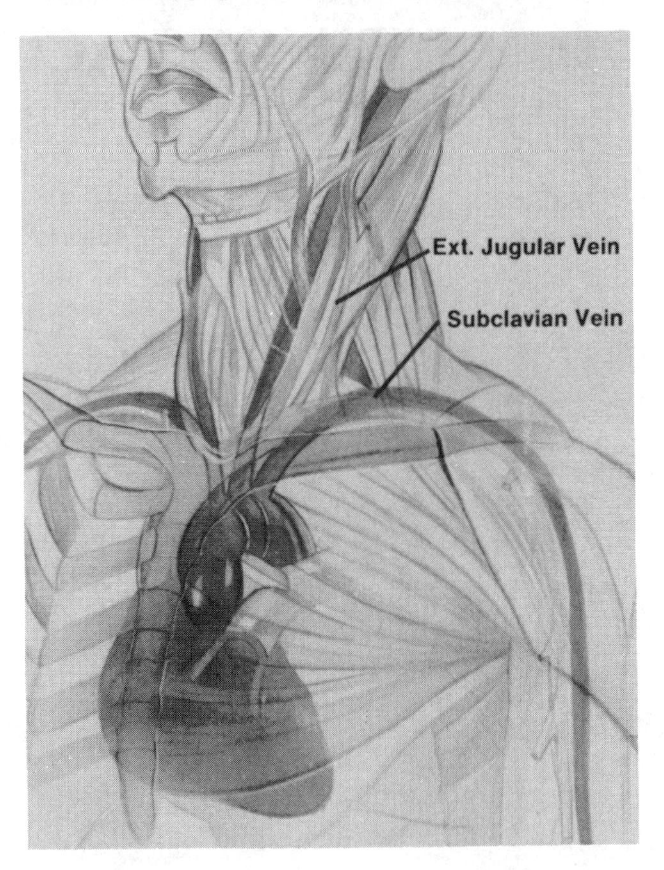

Shorter-term VADs are placed to exit from the external jugular or subclavian veins.

LONG-TERM CATHETERS

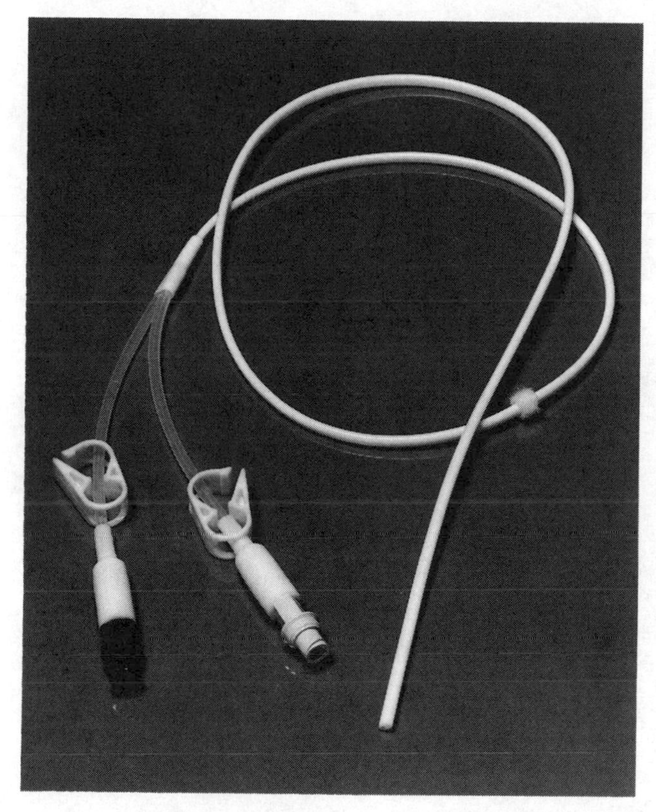

Tunneled VADs are long-term catheters that are surgically implanted, ending in the superior vena cava or right atrium of the heart. The access ports on these catheters are external. Depending on the catheter, the device can require clamping, frequent flushing and particular dressing changes to guard against infection. Examples of tunneled VADs are the Hickman, Broviac and Groshong catheters. Shown is a double-lumen Raff catheter. (For specific information on tunneled catheters, contact the manufacturer.)

Photo courtesy of Quinton Instrument Company, Seattle, WA.

IMPLANTED PORTS

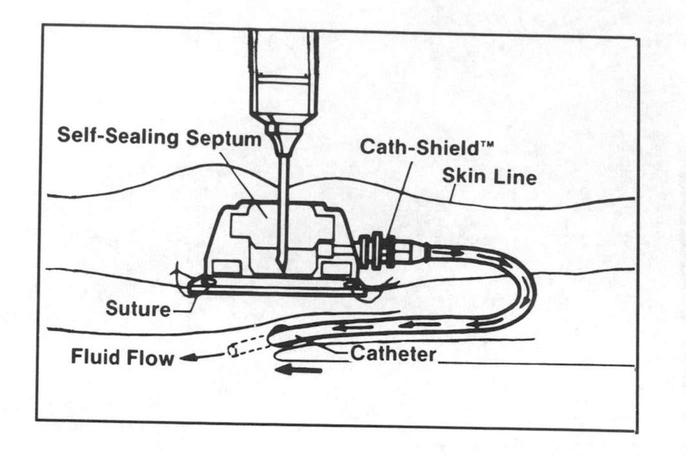

Implanted ports are long-term VADs surgically placed under the skin. They usually are accessed under the collarbone and terminate in the superior vena cava or the right atrium of the heart. The ports have a septum that can be accessed through the skin with a special Huber needle. These ports can be placed in other regions of the body to provide more direct access to that area. Shown is the Port-A-Cath.

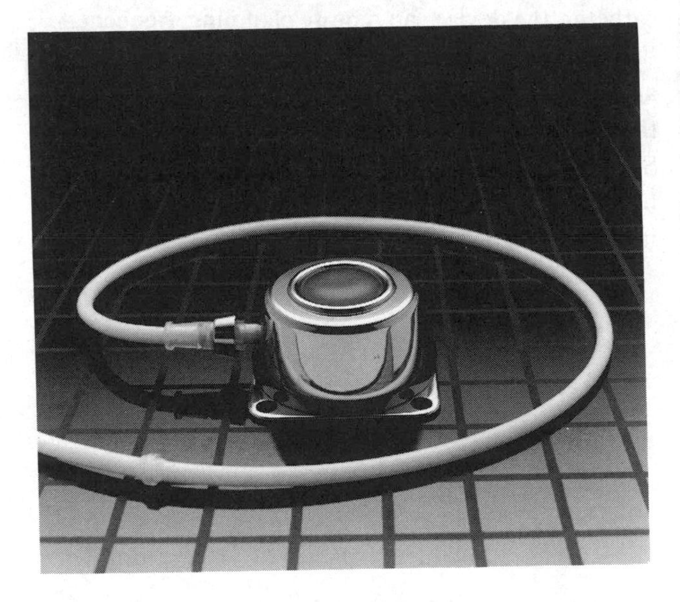

Drawing and photo reprinted with permission from Pharmacia Deltec, Inc., St. Paul, Minnesota.

IMPLANTED PUMPS
(Medtronic)

MEDTRONIC SYNCHROMED™ INFUSION PUMP

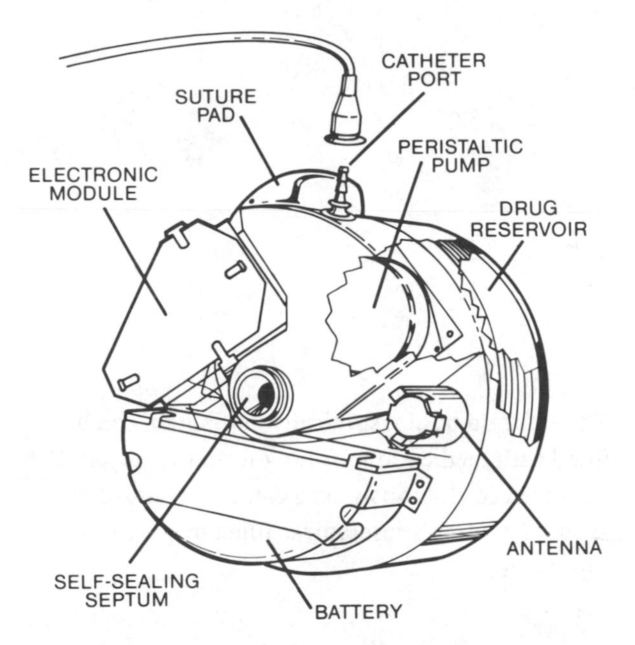

The Medtronic implantable pump, surgically placed, releases medication over a period of time, according to instructions from an external programmer. Medication is filled in the pump's reservoir, then released to the body site through a catheter.

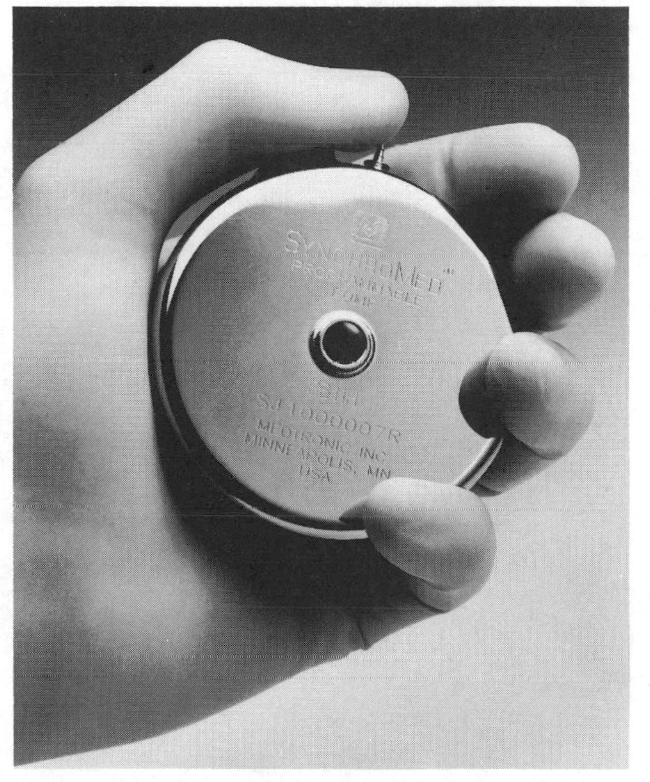

Drawing and photo reprinted with permission from Medtronic, Inc., Minneapolis, MN.

IMPLANTED PUMPS (INFUSAID)

The INFUSAID Pump

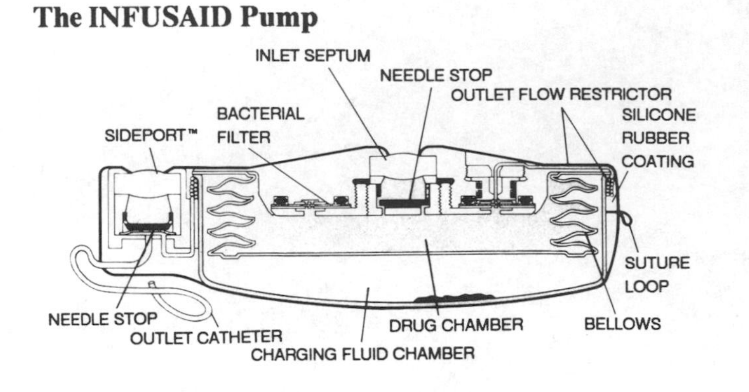

The Infusaid pump, surgically implanted, can be filled with medication for long-term therapy and delivered continuously via a catheter to selected sites. The pump's reservoir is filled by percutaneous injections.

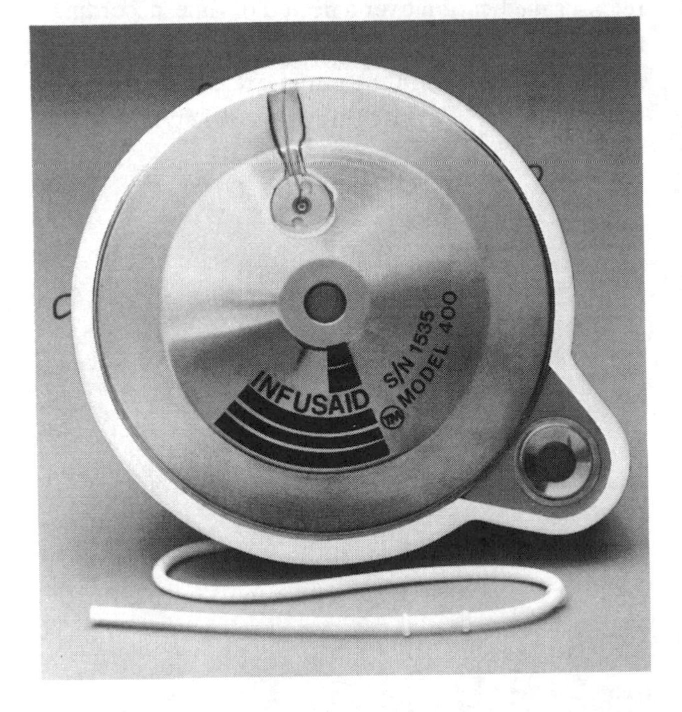

Photo and drawing reprinted with permission from Infusaid, Inc., Norwood, MA.

PICC LINE

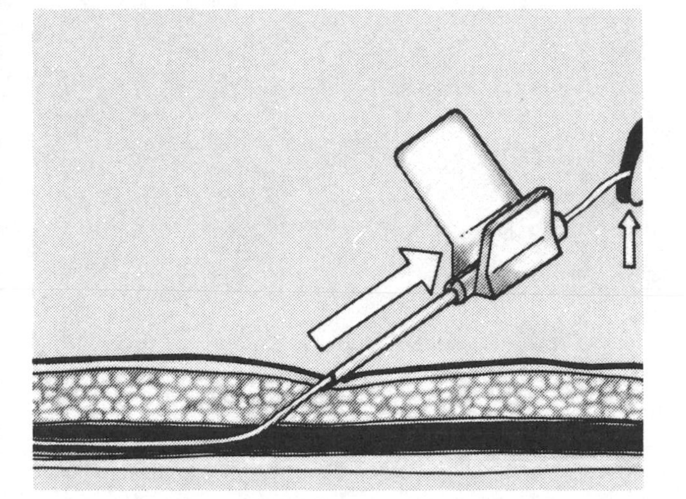

Peripherally Inserted Central Catheters can be placed without surgery, providing medium- to long-term access via a peripheral site. They are usually threaded up the arm: the basilic vein is the vein of choice. The distance that the catheter is threaded depends on the therapy to be infused and how long access is needed. Shown is the Per-Q-Cath PICC line.

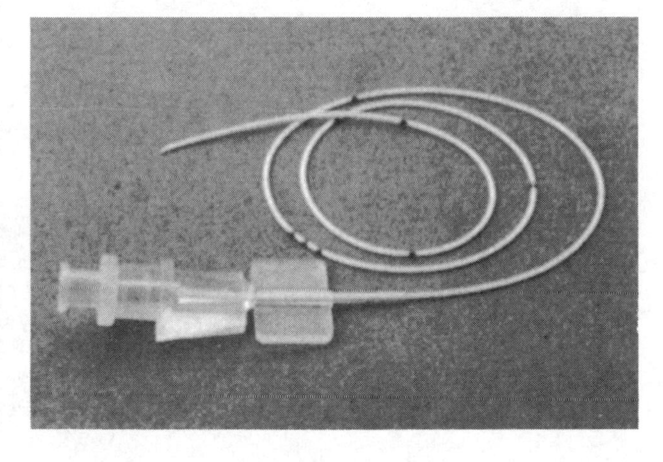

Drawing and photo reprinted with permission from Gesco, International, San Antonio, TX.

APPENDIX B

Performance Status Scales

Description: Karnofsky Scale	Karnofsky Scale (%)	Zubrod Scale (ECOG)	TNM Scale (AJC)	Description: AJC and ECOG Scales
No complaints; no evidence of disease Able to carry on normal activity; minor signs or symptoms of disease	100 90	0	H0	Normal activity
Some signs or symptoms of disease with effort Cares for self; unable to carry on normal activity or to do active work	80 70	1	H1	Symptoms of disease, but ambulatory and able to carry out activities of daily living
Requires occasional assistance but is able to carc for most personal needs Requires considerable assistance and frequent medical care	60 50	2	H2	Out of bed more than 50% of time; occasionally needs assistance
Disabled; requires special care and assistance Severely disabled; hospitalization indicated, although death not imminent	40 30	3	H3	In bed more than 50% of time; needs nursing care
Very sick; hospitalization necessary; requires active supportive treatment Moribund; fatal processes progressing rapidly	20 10	4	H4	Bedridden; may need hospitalization
Dead	0			

ECOG = Eastern Cooperative Oncology Group AJC = American Joint Commission for Cancer Staging and End Results Reporting

Source: Casciato, L. & Lowitz, B. B., (1983). *Manual of bedside oncology.* Boston: Little, Brown and Company. Reprinted with permission.

INDEX

A

Absolute granulocyte count (AGC), 60
ABVD administration, 76
Actinomycin D, 45-46
Adjuvant chemotherapy, 2, 79, 87
Administration,
  calculating doses of, 23
  checklist for, 22
  documentation on, 37
  dosages for, 79
  intraarterial route of, 32-33
  intracavitary/intraperitoneal route, 33-35
  intramuscular/subcutaneous routes of, 29
  intrathecal route of, 35
  intravenous route of, 29-32
  MOPP/ABVD, 76-77
  oral route of, 29
  outpatient, 81
  patient data for, 21-22
  pertinent laboratory data for, 22-23
  safe handling during, 35-37
  selecting route of, 23, 29
  ventricular reservoir, 35
  See also Chemotherapy
Adriamycin, 46-47
Adrucil (5-Fluorouracil) [5FU], 47-48
Adult Nomogram, 27
Alkylating agents, 15-16, 87
Allergic response, 69-70
Alopecia (hair loss), 64-66, 87
Anaphylaxis (allergic) response, 69-70
Anemia, 61
Anorexia, 66
Antiemetic, 87
Antimetabolites, 17, 87
Antineoplastic agents,
  cell cycle and, 10
  laboratory values altered by, 24-26
  vesicant/irritant, 68-69
Antitumor antibiotics, 17, 87
Arabinosid (ARA-C), 44-45
Asparaginase (ELSPAR) [L-asparaginase], 49-50

B

Basilic vein, 30
Benign, 2, 87
BiCNU (BCNU), 42-43
Bleomycin (Blenoxane), 41-42
Bone marrow suppression,
  anemia and, 61
  CSFs to fight, 79-80
  leukopenia and, 60-61
  nadir and, 61-62
  stomatitis (oral mucositis) and, 62, 88
  thrombocytopenia and, 61
Busulfan (Myleran), 42

C

Cancer cells,
  cell kill theory and, 11-12
  chemotherapy to prevent, 80
  growth of, 8-11
Carboplatin (Paraplatin), 77
Carboximide, 45
Carcinogen, 87
Carmustine (BiCNU) [BCNU]), 42-43
Catheters, 29-30, 32-33
CEENU (CCNU), 50
Cell cycle,
  antineoplastic agents and, 10
  described, 7-8, 87
Cell-cycle-phase-nonspecific agents, 9
Cell-cycle-phase-specific agents, 9
Cell generation cycle, 8
Cell growth rate, 8-11
Cell kill theory, 11-12
Cellular kinetics, 7
Central catheters, 29-30, 32-33
Cephalic vein, 30
Cerebrospinal fluid (CSF) tumors, 35
Cerubidine (Daunomycin, Rubidomycin), 46
Chemotherapeutic agents,
  administration of, 21-38
  alkylating, 15-16, 87
  antimetabolites, 17, 87

Asparaginase (ELSPAR) [L-asparaginase], 49-50
Bleomycin (Blenoxane), 41-42
Busulfan (Myleran), 42
Carmustine (BiCNU) [BCNU]), 42-43
Cisplatin (Platino) [DDP], 43
clinical trials of, 80
Cyclophosphamide (Cytoxan) [CTX], 44
Cytarabine (Cytosar-U) [Cytosine, Arabinosid, ARA-C], 44-45
Dacarbazine (Dtic-dome) [Imidazole, Carboximide], 45
Dactinomycin (Cosmegen) [Actinomycin D], 45-46
Daunorubicin (Cerubidine) [Daunomycin, Rubidomycin], 46
development of new, 77, 79
dosages of, 79
Doxorubicin Hydrochloride (Adriamycin), 46-47
drug classifications of, 15-18
emotogenic potential of, 65
Etoposide (VePesid) [VP-16], 47
extravasation (tissue loss) by, 68-69
Floxuridine (FUDR), 48
Fluorouracil (Adrucil) [5-Fluorouracil] [5FU], 47-48
Hydroxyurea (Hydrea), 48
Ifosfamide (IFEX) [Isophosphamide], 49
Lomustine (CEENU) [CCNU], 50
Mechlorethamine (Mustargen) [Nitrogen Mustard] [HN2], 50-51
Megestrol (Megace), 51
Mercaptopurine (Purinethol) [6MP], 54
Methotrexate (Mexate) [MTX], 51-52
Mitomycin (Mutamycin), 52
Mitoxantrone (Novantrone) [DHAD], 52-53
Plicamycin (Mithracin) [Mithramycin], 53
Prednisone (Deltasone, Orasone), 53-54
Procarbazine (Matulane), 54
safe handling of, 35-37
Tamoxifen (Nolvadex), 54-55
Thiotepa [Triethylene Thiophosphoramide], 55
Vinblastine (Velban), 55
Vincristine (Oncovin) [VCR], 56
Chemotherapy,
adjuvant, 2, 79, 87
alopecia (hair loss) caused by, 64-66
biology of, 7-12
cell kill theory and, 11-12
combination, 75-78, 87
effectiveness of, 2
goals of, 3-4
history of, 1
nausea/vomiting caused by, 64
outpatient administration of, 81
patient education on, 37-38
for preventing cancer, 80
secondary malignancy due to, 67
tumor sensitivity to, 3
vocabulary of, 2
Cisplatin (Platino) [DDP], 43
Clinical trials, 80
CNS hemorrhaging, 61
Colony stimulating factors (CSFs), 79-80
Combination chemotherapy, 75-78, 87
Complete response or remission (CR), 4
Constipation, 66
Control treatment, 4
Cosmegen (Actinomycin D), 45-46
Cure, 3-4
Cyclophosphamide (Cytoxan) [CTX], 44, 77, 79
Cytarabine (Cytosar-U) [Cytosine, Arabinosid, ARA-C], 44-45
Cytotoxic agents, 2, 87

D

Dacarbazine (Dtic-dome) [Imidazole, Carboximide], 45
Dactinomycin (Cosmegen) [Actinomycin D], 45-46
Daunomycin (Rubidomycin), 46
Daunorubicin (Cerubidine) [Daunomycin, Rubidomycin], 46
DDP, 43
Deltasone (Orasone), 53-54
DHAD, 52-53
Diarrhea, 67
Documentation,
administration, 37
extravasation, 70
Dosages, 79
Doxorubicin Hydrochloride (Adriamycin), 46-47

Drug classifications,
  alkylating agents, 15-16
  antimetabolites, 17
  antitumor antibiotics, 17
  hormones, 18
  miscellaneous agents, 18
  nitrosoureas, 18
  plant alkaloids, 17-18

E

ELSPAR (L-asparaginase), 49-50
Emotogenic potential, 65
Eosinophils, 23
Etoposide (VePesid) [VP-16], 47
Extravasation record, 70
Extravasation (tissue loss), 68-69, 87

F

5-Fluorouracil (5FU), 47-48
Floxuridine (FUDR), 48
Fluorouracil (Adrucil) [5-Fluorouracil] [5FU], 47-48

G

GI hemorrhaging, 61
Gompertzian function, 12
Gonadal dysfunction, 67-68
Granulocyte colony-stimulating factor (G-CSF), 79
Granulocyte/macrophage colony-stimulating factor (GM-CSF), 79
Granulocytes, 23
Growth factors, 87
Growth fraction, 87

H

Hair loss (alopecia), 64-66, 73
Hemorrhaging, 61
HN2, 50-51
Hormones, 18
Hydroxyurea (Hydrea), 48

I

Ifosfamide (IFEX) [Isophosphamide], 49, 77, 79
Imidazole (Carboximide), 45
Immunotherapy, 77
Implanted ports, 33
Informed consent, 35
Interferon, 77
Intraarterial route, 32-33
Intracavitary route, 33-35
Intramuscular (IM) route, 29
Intraperitoneal (IP) route, 33-35
Intrathecal route, 35
Intravenous (IV) route, 29-32
Irritant antineoplastic drugs, 69, 87

L

Laboratory data,
  altered by antineoplastic agents, 24-26
  myelosuppression, 63
  patient, 22-23
  suggesting nephrotoxic effects, 67
L-asparaginase, 49-50
Leukopenia, 60-61

M

Macrophage colony-stimulating factor (M-CSF), 79
Malignant, 2, 87
Matulane, 54
Mechlorethamine (Mustargen) [Nitrogen Mustard] [HN2], 50-51
Median antebrachial vein, 30
Median basilic vein, 30
Median cephalic vein, 30
Megestrol (Megace), 51
Mercaptopurine (Purinethol) [6MP], 54
Mesna (Mesnex), 77
Metastasize, 2, 87
Methotrexate (Mexate) [MTX], 51-52
Meylosuppression, 63
  See also Nadir
Miscellaneous agents, 18
Mithracin (Mithramycin), 53
Mitomycin (Mutamycin), 52
Mitoxantrone (Novantrone) [DHAD], 52-53
MOPP administration, 76-77

Mustargen (Nitrogen Mustard) [HN2], 50-51
Myleran, 42

N

Nadir, 61-62, 76, 87
National Cancer Institute, 1
National Study Commission on Cytotoxic Exposure, 35
Nausea, 64
Neoplasm, 2, 87
Nephrotoxic effects, 67
Neutropenia, 87
Neutrophils, 23
Nitrogen Mustard (HN2), 50-51
Nitrosoureas, 18, 87
Nolvadex, 54-55
Nomograms,
  adult, 27
  pediatric, 28
Novantrone (DHAD), 52-53
Nurses,
  anaphylaxis (allergic) guidelines for, 69-70
  clinical trial role of, 80
  cytotoxic agents handling guidelines for, 35-37
  documenting administration by, 37
  informed consent role of, 35
  patient education role of, 37-38
  side effect management by, 59-71

O

Ommaya reservoir, 36
Oncovin [VCR], 56
Oral candidiasis, 62
Oral mucositis, 62
Oral route, 29
Orasone, 53-54
OSHA guidelines (handling cytotoxic agents), 35-37
Outpatient administration, 81

P

Pain management, 71
Palliation, 4, 87
Paraplatin, 77
Partial response (PR), 4
Patients,
  alopecia (hair loss) in, 64-66, 87
  anaphylaxis (allergic) response by, 69-70
  anorexia/weight loss in, 66
  bone marrow suppression in, 60-62
  chemotherapy administration to, 21-22
  clinical trial, 80
  constipation in, 66
  diarrhea in, 67
  educating the, 37-38
  extravasation (tissue loss) in, 68-69, 87
  gonadal dysfunction (sterility) in, 67-68
  informed consent of, 35
  laboratory data on, 22-23
  nausea/vomiting in, 64
  nephrotoxic effects in, 67
  pain of, 71
  psychosocial issues of, 71
  secondary malignancy in, 67
  stomatitis in, 62
  vascular access device assessment of, 34
Pediatric nomogram, 28
Peripheral veins, 29
Plant alkaloids, 17-18
Platelet counts, 61
Platinol (DDP), 43
Plicamycin (Mithracin) [Mithramycin], 53
Prednisone (Deltasone, Orasone), 53-54
Procarbazine (Matulane), 54
Progression, 4
Proliferate, 2
Psychosocial issues, 71
Purinethol (6MP), 54

R

Radiation, 77
Renal status, 23
Rubidomycin, 46

S

Secondary malignancy, 67
Silastic atrial catheters, 32-33
6MP, 54
Small-gauge central venous catheters, 32-33

Solid tumor, 2
Stable disease (SD), 4
Sterility, 67-68
Stomatitis (oral mucositis), 62, 88
Subcutaneous (SC) route, 29

T

Tamoxifen (Nolvadex), 54-55
Thiotepa [Triethylene Thiophosphoramide], 55
Thrombocytopenia, 61, 88
Tumor doubling time, 88
Tumors,
  of cerebrospinal fluid (CSF), 35
  defining, 2, 88
  response criteria of, 4
  sensitivity classification of, 3
Two-syringe technique, 30-31

V

Valsalva maneuver, 88
VCR, 56
Venipuncture sites,
  administration through, 31
  arm, 29
  on dorsum of hand, 30
Venous access devices (VAD),
  patient assessment for, 34
  using, 29-30, 32-33
Ventricular reservoir,
  described, 35
  Ommaya, 36
VePesid (VP-16), 47
Vesicant antineoplastic drugs, 68-69, 88
Vinblastine (Velban), 55
Vinca alkaloids, 17-18, 88
Vincristine (Oncovin) [VCR], 56
Vomiting, 64

W

Weight loss, 66
White blood cell (WBC) count,
  AGC and, 60
  described, 23
  MOPP/ABVD administration and, 76

PRE-TEST ANSWER KEY

BASICS OF CANCER CHEMOTHERAPY

1. A Chapter 1
2. B Chapter 2
3. A Chapter 6
4. D Chapter 4
5. B Chapter 4
6. B Chapter 6
7. D Chapter 7
8. C Chapter 5
9. B Chapter 6
10. B Chapter 6